Oral Candidosis

Edvaldo Antonio Ribeiro Rosa
Editor

Oral Candidosis

Physiopathology, Decision Making, and Therapeutics

Springer

Editor
Edvaldo Antonio Ribeiro Rosa
School of Health and Biosciences
Pontifical Catholic University of Paraná
Curitiba, Paraná
Brazil

ISBN 978-3-662-47193-7 ISBN 978-3-662-47194-4 (eBook)
DOI 10.1007/978-3-662-47194-4

Library of Congress Control Number: 2015949091

Springer Heidelberg New York Dordrecht London

Printed on acid-free paper

Springer-Verlag GmbH Berlin Heidelberg is part of Springer Science+Business Media
(www.springer.com)

Contents

Contributors

Luciana Reis Azevedo Alanis Graduate Program in Dentistry, School of Health and Biosciences, Pontifícia Universidade Católica do Paraná, Curitiba, Brazil

Patrícia Vida Cassi Bettega, DDS, MSc School of Health and Biosciences, Pontifícia Universidade Católica do Paraná, Curitiba, Brazil

Patrícia Carlos Caldeira, DDS, MSc, PhD Department of Oral Surgery and Oral Pathology, School of Dentistry, Universidade Federal de Minas Gerais, Belo Horizonte, MG, Brazil

Soraya de A. Berti Couto Stomatology, School of Health and Biosciences, Pontifícia Universidade Católica do Paraná, Curitiba, Brazil

Altair A. Del Bel Cury Department of Prosthodontics and Periodontology, Piracicaba Dental School, State University of Campinas, Piracicaba, SP, Brazil

Wander José da Silva Department of Prosthodontics and Periodontology, Piracicaba Dental School, State University of Campinas, Piracicaba, SP, Brazil

Soluete Oliveira da Silva Department of Stomatology, University of Passo Fundo, Passo Fundo, Rio Grande do Sul, Brazil

Bethânia Molin Giaretta De Carli, MSc Department of Oral and Maxillofacial Surgery, University of Passo Fundo, Passo Fundo, Rio Grande do Sul, Brazil

João Paulo De Carli Department of Stomatology, University of Passo Fundo, Passo Fundo, Rio Grande do Sul, Brazil

Antonio Adilson Soares de Lima Faculty of Dentistry, Federal University of Paraná, Curitiba, Brazil

Mariela Dutra Gontijo de Moura, DDS, MSc, PhD Department of Oral Surgery and Pathology, School of Dentistry, Universidade Federal de Minas Gerais, Belo Horizonte, MG, Brazil

Andréa Araújo de Vasconcellos Department of Restorative Dentistry, Federal University of Juiz de Fora, Juiz de Fora, MG, Brazil

Renata Serignoli Francisconi Department of Physiology and Pathology, Araraquara Dental School, State University of São Paulo, São Paulo, Brazil

Letícia Machado Gonçalves Faculty of Dentistry, CEUMA University, São Luiz do Maranhão, MG, Brazil

Ana Maria Trindade Grégio, BPharm, MSc, PhD School of Health and Biosciences, Pontifícia Universidade Católica do Paraná, Curitiba, PR, Brazil

Cristiane Yumi Koga Ito Institute of Science and Technology, Oral Biopathology Program and Department of Environmental Engineering, Universidade Estadual Paulista/UNESP, São José dos Campos, Brazil

Ruwan Duminda Jayasinghe Department of Oral Medicine and Periodontology, Faculty of Dental Sciences, University of Peradeniya, Peradeniya, Sri Lanka

Aline Cristina Batista Rodrigues Johann, DDS, MSc, PhD School of Health and Biosciences, Pontifícia Universidade Católica do Paraná, Curitiba, PR, Brazil

Maria Salete Sandini Linden Department of Implantology, Post-graduate Program in Dentistry, University of Passo Fundo, Passo Fundo, Rio Grande do Sul, Brazil

Maria Ângela Naval Machado Faculty of Dentistry, Federal University of Paraná, Curitiba, Brazil

Lindsay E. O'Donnell Glasgow Dental School, School of Medicine, College of Medical, Veterinary and Life Sciences, University of Glasgow, Glasgow, UK

Daniel Freitas Alves Pereira Institute of Science and Technology, Oral Biopathology Graduate Program, Universidade Estadual Paulista/UNESP, São José dos Campos, Brazil

Gordon Ramage Glasgow Dental School, School of Medicine, College of Medical, Veterinary and Life Sciences, University of Glasgow, Glasgow, UK

Mariana Rinaldi, DDS, MSc School of Health and Biosciences, Pontifícia Universidade Católica do Paraná, Curitiba, Brazil

Douglas Robertson Glasgow Dental School, School of Medicine, College of Medical, Veterinary and Life Sciences, University of Glasgow, Glasgow, UK

Edvaldo Antonio Ribeiro Rosa School of Health and Biosciences, Xenobiotics Research Unit, The Pontifical Catholic University of Paraná, Curitiba, Brazil

Jorgiana Sangalli Institute of Science and Technology, Oral Biopathology Graduate Program, Universidade Estadual Paulista/UNESP, São José dos Campos, Brazil

Chaminda Jayampath Seneviratne Oral Sciences, Faculty of Dentistry, National University of Singapore, Singapore

Paulo Henrique Couto Souza Stomatology, School of Health and Biosciences, Pontifícia Universidade Católica do Paraná, Curitiba, Brazil

Denise M. Palomari Spolidorio Department of Physiology and Pathology, Araraquara Dental School, State University of São Paulo, São Paulo, Brazil

Luís Carlos Spolidorio Department of Physiology and Pathology, Araraquara School of Dentistry, Sao Paulo State University (UNESP), Araraquara, SP, Brazil

Micheline Sandini Trentin Department of Implantology, Post-graduate Program in Dentistry, University of Passo Fundo, Passo Fundo, Rio Grande do Sul, Brazil

Flávia Fusco Veiga, DDS, MSc, School of Health and Biosciences, Pontifícia Universidade Católica do Paraná, Curitiba, Brazil

Angélica Zanata Department of Stomatology, University of Passo Fundo, Passo Fundo, Rio Grande do Sul, Brazil

Oral Candidosis Epidemiology 1

Edvaldo Antonio Ribeiro Rosa

Abstract

Oral candidosis (syn. oral candidiasis; OC) is considered the most common mycosis occurring in human beings. *Candida* spp. involved on OC are widely spread among people from different parts of the globe.

Differently from other microbes, the mere isolation of *Candida* from intraoral surfaces is not interpreted as a predictive signal for disease. The commensal status of such fungal genus has been evaluated along the years and according to different authors, 54–71.4 % of healthy individuals from diverse populations may carry such yeasts without any symptom. Although high counts of yeast cells in saliva may be interpreted as a suggestive signal of candidosis, not always it will occur.

Oral candidosis (syn. oral candidiasis; OC) is considered the most common mycosis occurring in human beings. *Candida* spp. involved on OC are widely spread among people from different parts of the globe.

Differently from other microbes, the mere isolation of *Candida* from intraoral surfaces is not interpreted as a predictive signal for disease. The commensal status of such fungal genus has been evaluated along the years and according to different authors, 54–71.4 % of healthy individuals from diverse populations may carry such yeasts without any symptom (Hauman et al. 1993; Darwazeh and al-Bashir 1995; Kindelan et al. 1998; Blignaut et al. 2002). Although high counts of yeast cells in saliva may be interpreted as a suggestive signal of candidosis, not always it will occur. Akpan and Morgan (2002) have compiled data concerning to carrier status of individuals from different risk groups and stated that in the general population, carriage rates have been reported to range from 20 to 75 % without any symptoms. According to them, the incidence of *Candida* isolated from the oral cavity (not related to OC episodes) has been reported to be 45 % in neonates, 45–65 % of healthy children, 30–45 % of healthy adults, 50–65 % of people who wear removable dentures, 65–88 % in those residing in acute and long-term care facilities, 90 % of patients with acute leukemia undergoing chemotherapy, and 95 % of patients with HIV.

E.A.R. Rosa
School of Health and Biosciences, Xenobiotics Research Unit, The Pontifical Catholic University of Paraná, Curitiba, Brazil
e-mail: edvaldo.rosa@pucpr.br

E.A.R. Rosa (ed.), *Oral Candidosis: Physiopathology, Decision Making, and Therapeutics*,
DOI 10.1007/978-3-662-47194-4_1

Albeit the above statement, OC occurs when some predisposing conditions favor the fungal pathogenic shift.

Regarding to age, there is a medical maxim that says "oral thrush (syn. pseudomembranous candidosis, moniliasis) is common in the very young, the very old, or the very sick".

Oral thrush is a disease affecting around 1 in 20 babies. The Centers for Disease Control and Prevention estimates that OC is seen in between 5 and 7 % of babies less than 1 month old (CDC 2013). Premature babies (born before 37 weeks) have an increased risk of developing oral thrush. There is a consensus among pediatricians and pediatric dentists that oral thrush may occur in infants up to 2 years old.

People belonging to the second group in the aphorism (very old people) are more prone to develop OC due to their compromised health conditions and, for a great group of them, to the fact that they wear dentures. Elderly, almost always, implies in a diminishing of immune status with age-related high expression of TGF-β and low elastase and salivary peroxidase activities. Also, negative modulating receptors expression on salivary neutrophils may occur (Gasparoto et al., 2012). Add to that, the fact that elder people experience a decrease and a functional impairment in the population of circulating T cells (Girard et al., 1977).

Other comorbidities and conditions typical of such population as diabetes, hypertension, dehydration, undernutrition, and medicine intake to treat anxiety or depression lead to severe reductions in the salivary production, incurring in high predisposition to convert saprophytic yeasts into opportunistic pathogens.

Epidemiological data show that 65–84.1 % of elder denture wearers may harbor *Candida* spp. in their mouths (Budtz-Jorgensen et al., 1975; de Resende et al., 2006). Dentures per se constitute a predisposing factor for candidosis, once the acrylic surfaces act as a fungal reservoir. Also, broken and loosely adapted dentures may cause attrition-related lesions in which the fungus develops more promptly.

The deleterious habit of cigarette smoking is clearly recognized as a predisposing factor for OC, and the heavy cigarette consumption are associated with predisposition to some complications. The smoking habit may provoke increased oral epithelial keratinization and subsequent enhancement of hydrophobicity, which may predispose the smoker to higher oral yeast colonization (Williams et al., 1999).

It was demonstrated that constituents of cigarette smoke may increase fungal virulence attributes (Baboni et al., 2009, 2010). Soysa and Ellepola (2005) compiled data from various studies and stated that cigarette smoking provokes increments in oral candidal carriage in smokers. Complications like candidal leukoplakia (Arendorf et al., 1983; Daftary et al., 1972) are more commonly found occurring in smokers than in nonsmokers. Chronic hyperplastic candidosis can be solved by suppressing tobacco consumption (Holmstrup and Bessermann 1983).

Although less remarkable than those high casuistic values for candidal vaginitis (25–70 %) or intestinal *Candida* overgrowth (55.9–63.2 %) after antibiotic therapy, OC is a commonly reported side effect. However, few studies have tried to determine the incidence of such predisposing conditions for OC.

The reduction in salivary flow rate is universally considered as one of the most important predisposing factor for oral candidal increments and candidosis. Some conditions can determine or contribute to such events. Salivary gland hypofunction may be a result of (i) enhanced sympathetic drive during prolonged anxiety events; (ii) age-related dehydration, diabetes, or inaccessibility to water; (iii) isolated or polypharmacy iatrogenic action of anticholinergics (atropine, atropinics, and hyoscine), central-acting psychoactive agents (antidepressants, phenothiazines, benzodiazepines, and antihistamines), drugs acting on sympathetic system (sympathomimetics, alpha-1 antagonists, alfa-2 agonists and beta-blockers), cytotoxic drugs, diuretics, opioids, methamphetamine, heroin, and correlates, among other medicines and illegal drugs; (iv) prolonged diarrhea; (v) renal failure; and (vi) Sjögren's syndrome; (vii) radiotherapy to treat head/neck cancer; among others.

As this condition may be caused by numberless etiologic factors, the epidemiology of hyposalivation-related OC is somehow difficult to be established. Among people suffering from Sjögren's syndrome, OC may achieve 87 % of patients (Yan et al., 2011). It has been reported that 55.2 % of patients with cancer in the head/neck region who were in a radiotherapy regimen experienced OC during the course of the treatment (Deng et al., 2010).

Besides periodontal diseases and caries, the negligence in oral cleansing also can drive to candidosis. This negligence is especially markedly in some risk groups as elders, drug addicts, and hospitalized patients.

Despite the increase in predisposition to OC in denture wearers, per se, factors as educational status, level of income, dental visiting frequency, denture conditions, brushing methods, and brushing frequency are determinants of OC. Positive relationships can be observed between poor denture hygiene habits and denture-related stomatitis, in up to 44 % of patients (Evren et al., 2011). Some patients merely wash their prosthesis with water or just with a toothbrush.

According to the Recovery Organization, an estimated 40–60 % of those addicted to drugs face addiction relapse (Recovery.org 2013). The low self-esteem led such individuals to neglect their appearance and hygiene. It has been demonstrated that 10.9 % of polydrug users attended in a specialized clinic in Madrid, Spain, presented angular cheilitis (Mateos-Moreno et al., 2013), a condition commonly found in people with nutritional deficiencies (especially, folate, iron, or vitamin B2), poorly maintained dentures, or immunosuppression.

Poor oral hygiene also is critical for hospitalized patients. A survey conducted in a Brazilian hospital revealed that oral hygiene is more commonly associated to age than to physical disability (Carrilho Neto et al., 2011). Involved investigators reported that 69 % of patients presented poor oral hygiene and 19.6 % presented OC. Some other complications as coma (Cecon et al., 2010), cancer (Meurman and Gronroos 2010; Davies et al., 2008), dentures (Tosello et al., 2008), or immunosuppression (Palmason et al., 2011) tend to increase the possibility of institutionalized patients to develop OC.

People suffering from central nervous system diseases, mainly those receiving heavy psychotropic medications with anticholinergic effects, are more prone to experience OC once hyposalivation may occur as a result of the burden of combined drugs as chlorpromazine, benztropine, lithium, and risperidone (Stevens 2007). In some cases, patients with deep nervous disorders (e.g., dementia) require accessory treatment to attenuate OC that occurs (Lloyd-Williams 1996).

Other group of patients that requires special dedicated attention is the terminally ill patients. OC is common in advanced cancer cases occurring in 31–70 % or 83 % of patients and clearly affecting the quality of their remaining life (Aldred et al., 1991; Ball et al., 1998; Butticaz et al., 2003). As most of those patients are aged and wear dentures, a high proportion of them present diverse variants of OC, including angular cheilitis (Chaushu et al., 2000). Molecular methods based on fungal DNA fingerprinting revealed that antifungal treatment in this patient group fails to eradicate the original *Candida* sp. strain, thereby allowing recolonization of the oral cavity (Wilson et al., 2001).

There are no doubts that the most well-known predisposing factor to OC is the immunosuppressant effect of human immunodeficiency virus (HIV) in AIDS patients.

Before the advent of the highly active antiretroviral therapy (HAART) era in 2000–2001, oral candidoses were common comorbidities occurring in a variable range of 50–52 % (Schulten et al., 1989; Morace et al., 1990; Ramirez et al., 1990) to 94 % (Tukutuku et al., 1990) of HIV-infected individuals. HAART has produced an impressive decline in the incidence of opportunistic infections in HIV-infected adults and children becoming uncommon. In certain cases, such prevalence has dropped to as low values as 1.87 % (Gona et al., 2006). However, in some localities, the addicts' ignorance or the inaccessibility to medication imply high casuistic of OC (Solomon et al., 2008; Evans et al., 2012; Pattrapornnan and Derouen 2013; Zhang et al., 2009) even in industrialized countries (Tappuni and Fleming 2001; Tami-Maury et al. 2011).

A particular predisposing factor for OC is diabetes mellitus. It is estimated that 15.1 % of insulin-dependent diabetes mellitus (IDDM) (Guggenheimer et al., 2000) and 24 % of type-2 diabetes are prone to OC (Bajaj et al., 2012). Indeed, the diabetic patient presents various predisposing conditions that corroborate to OC occurring as hyposalivation, impaired local immune response, higher salivary glucose concentration; many of them wear dentures, etc.

Of significant importance, literature reveals that there is a significant higher obtaining of *Candida albicans* than other *Candida* spp. in positive oral harvestings. Such result is perceptible in both healthy carriers and ill individuals (Obladen 2012; Calcaterra et al., 2013; Castro et al., 2013; Gammelsrud et al., 2011; Manas et al., 2012; Rautemaa and Ramage 2011; Santiwongkarn et al., 2012; Westbrook et al., 2013). The pathogenic/virulent attributes of *Candida* spp. as well as their role in the development of OC are discussed in other chapters of this book.

References

Akpan A, Morgan R (2002) Oral candidiasis. Postgrad Med J 78(922):455–459

Aldred MJ, Addy M, Bagg J, Finlay I (1991) Oral health in the terminally ill: a cross-sectional pilot survey. Spec Care Dentist 11(2):59–62

Arendorf TM, Walker DM, Kingdom RJ, Roll JR, Newcombe RG (1983) Tobacco smoking and denture wearing in oral candidal leukoplakia. Br Dent J 155(10): 340–343

Baboni FB, Barp D, Izidoro AC, Samaranayake LP, Rosa EA (2009) Enhancement of Candida albicans virulence after exposition to cigarette mainstream smoke. Mycopathologia 168(5):227–235. doi:10.1007/s11046-009-9217-5

Baboni FB, Guariza Filho O, Moreno AN, Rosa EA (2010) Influence of cigarette smoke condensate on cardiogenic and candidal biofilm formation on orthodontic materials. Am J Orthodontics Dentofacial Orthopedics 138(4):427–434. doi:10.1016/j.ajodo.2009.05.023

Bajaj S, Prasad S, Gupta A, Singh VB (2012) Oral manifestations in type-2 diabetes and related complications. Indian J Endocrinol Metab 16(5):777–779. doi:10.4103/2230-8210.100673

Ball K, Sweeney MP, Baxter WP, Bagg J (1998) Fluconazole sensitivities of Candida species isolated from the mouths of terminally ill cancer patients. Am J Hosp Palliat Care 15(6):315–319

Blignaut E, Pujol C, Lockhart S, Joly S, Soll DR (2002) Ca3 fingerprinting of Candida albicans isolates from human immunodeficiency virus-positive and healthy individuals reveals a new clade in South Africa. J Clin Microbiol 40(3):826–836

Budtz-Jorgensen E, Stenderup A, Grabowski M (1975) An epidemiologic study of yeasts in elderly denture wearers. Community Dent Oral Epidemiol 3(3):115–119

Butticaz G, Zulian GB, Preumont M, Budtz-Jorgensen E (2003) Evaluation of a nystatin-containing mouth rinse for terminally ill patients in palliative care. J Palliat Care 19(2):95–99

Calcaterra R, Pasquantonio G, Vitali LA, Nicoletti M, Di Girolamo M, Mirisola C, Prenna M, Condo R, Baggi L (2013) Occurrence of Candida species colonization in a population of denture-wearing immigrants. Int J Immunopathol Pharmacol 26(1):239–246

Carrilho Neto A, De Paula RS, Sant'ana AC, Passanezi E (2011) Oral health status among hospitalized patients. Int J Dent Hyg 9(1):21–29. doi:10.1111/j.1601-5037.2009.00423.x

Castro LA, Alvarez MI, Martinez E (2013) Pseudomembranous candidiasis in HIV/AIDS patients in Cali, Colombia. Mycopathologia 175(1-2):91–98. doi:10.1007/s11046-012-9593-0

CDC (2013) CDC 24/7: saving lives. Protecting People™. Centers for Disease Control and Prevention. http://www.cdc.gov/fungal/diseases/candidiasis/thrush/statistics.html

Cecon F, Ferreira LE, Rosa RT, Gursky LC, de Paula e Carvalho A, Samaranayake LP, Rosa EA (2010) Time-related increase of staphylococci, Enterobacteriaceae and yeasts in the oral cavities of comatose patients. J Microbiol Immunol Infect = Wei mian yu gan ran za zhi 43(6):457–463. doi: 10.1016/S1684-1182(10)60071-0

Chaushu G, Bercovici M, Dori S, Waller A, Taicher S, Kronenberg J, Talmi YP (2000) Salivary flow and its relation with oral symptoms in terminally ill patients. Cancer 88(5):984–987

Daftary DK, Mehta FS, Gupta PC, Pindborg JJ (1972) The presence of Candida in 723 oral leukoplakias among Indian villagers. Scand J Dent Res 80(1):75–79

Darwazeh AM, al-Bashir A (1995) Oral candidal flora in healthy infants. J Oral Pathol Med 24(8):361–364

Davies AN, Brailsford SR, Beighton D, Shorthose K, Stevens VC (2008) Oral candidosis in community-based patients with advanced cancer. J Pain Symptom Manage 35(5):508–514. doi:10.1016/j.jpainsymman.2007.07.005

de Resende MA, de Sousa LV, de Oliveira RC, Koga-Ito CY, Lyon JP (2006) Prevalence and antifungal susceptibility of yeasts obtained from the oral cavity of elderly individuals. Mycopathologia 162(1):39–44. doi:10.1007/s11046-006-0029-6

Deng Z, Kiyuna A, Hasegawa M, Nakasone I, Hosokawa A, Suzuki M (2010) Oral candidiasis in patients receiving radiation therapy for head and neck can-

cer. Otolaryngol–Head Neck Surg 143(2):242–247. doi:10.1016/j.otohns.2010.02.003
Evans D, Maskew M, Sanne I (2012) Increased risk of mortality and loss to follow-up among HIV-positive patients with oropharyngeal candidiasis and malnutrition before antiretroviral therapy initiation: a retrospective analysis from a large urban cohort in Johannesburg, South Africa. Oral Surg Oral Med Oral Pathol Oral Radiol 113(3):362–372. doi:10.1016/j.oooo.2011.09.004
Evren BA, Uludamar A, Iseri U, Ozkan YK (2011) The association between socioeconomic status, oral hygiene practice, denture stomatitis and oral status in elderly people living different residential homes. Arch Gerontol Geriatr 53(3):252–257. doi:10.1016/j.archger.2010.12.016
Gammelsrud KW, Sandven P, Hoiby EA, Sandvik L, Brandtzaeg P, Gaustad P (2011) Colonization by Candida in children with cancer, children with cystic fibrosis, and healthy controls. Clin Microbiol Infect 17(12):1875–1881. doi:10.1111/j.1469-0691.2011.03528.x
Gasparoto TH, Sipert CR, de Oliveira CE, Porto VC, Santos CF, Campanelli AP, Lara VS (2012) Salivary immunity in elderly individuals presented with Candida-related denture stomatitis. Gerodontology 29(2):e331–e339. doi:10.1111/j.1741-2358.2011.00476.x
Girard JP, Paychere M, Cuevas M, Fernandes B (1977) Cell-mediated immunity in an ageing population. Clin Exp Immunol 27(1):85–91
Gona P, Van Dyke RB, Williams PL, Dankner WM, Chernoff MC, Nachman SA, Seage GR 3rd (2006) Incidence of opportunistic and other infections in HIV-infected children in the HAART era. JAMA 296(3):292–300. doi:10.1001/jama.296.3.292
Guggenheimer J, Moore PA, Rossie K, Myers D, Mongelluzzo MB, Block HM, Weyant R, Orchard T (2000) Insulin-dependent diabetes mellitus and oral soft tissue pathologies: II. Prevalence and characteristics of Candida and Candidal lesions. Oral Surg Oral Med Oral Pathol Oral Radiol Endod 89(5):570–576
Hauman CH, Thompson IO, Theunissen F, Wolfaardt P (1993) Oral carriage of Candida in healthy and HIV-seropositive persons. Oral Surg Oral Med Oral Pathol 76(5):570–572
Holmstrup P, Bessermann M (1983) Clinical, therapeutic, and pathogenic aspects of chronic oral multifocal candidiasis. Oral Surg Oral Med Oral Pathol 56(4):388–395
Kindelan SA, Yeoman CM, Douglas CW, Franklin C (1998) A comparison of intraoral Candida carriage in Sjogren's syndrome patients with healthy xerostomic controls. Oral Surg Oral Med Oral Pathol Oral Radiol Endod 85(2):162–167
Lloyd-Williams M (1996) An audit of palliative care in dementia. Eur J Cancer Care 5(1):53–55
Manas A, Cerezo L, de la Torre A, Garcia M, Alburquerque H, Ludena B, Ruiz A, Perez A, Escribano A, Manso A, Glaria LA, Grupo de Investigacion Clinica en Oncologia R (2012) Epidemiology and prevalence of oropharyngeal candidiasis in Spanish patients with head and neck tumors undergoing radiotherapy treatment alone or in combination with chemotherapy. Clin Transl Oncol 14(10):740–746. doi:10.1007/s12094-012-0861-8
Mateos-Moreno MV, Del-Rio-Highsmith J, Rioboo-Garcia R, Sola-Ruiz MF, Celemin-Vinuela A (2013) Dental profile of a community of recovering drug addicts: biomedical aspects. Retrospective cohort study. Med Oral Patol Oral Cir Bucal 18(4):e671–e679
Meurman JH, Gronroos L (2010) Oral and dental health care of oral cancer patients: hyposalivation, caries and infections. Oral Oncol 46(6):464–467. doi:10.1016/j.oraloncology.2010.02.025
Morace G, Tamburrini E, Manzara S, Antinori A, Maiuro G, Dettori G (1990) Epidemiological and clinical aspects of mycoses in patients with AIDS-related pathologies. Eur J Epidemiol 6(4):398–403
Obladen M (2012) Thrush – nightmare of the foundling hospitals. Neonatology 101(3):159–165. doi:10.1159/000329879
Palmason S, Marty FM, Treister NS (2011) How do we manage oral infections in allogeneic stem cell transplantation and other severely immunocompromised patients? Oral Maxillofac Surg Clin North Am 23(4):579–599. doi:10.1016/j.coms.2011.07.012, vii
Pattrapornnan P, Derouen TA (2013) Associations of periodontitis and oral manifestations with CD4 counts in human immunodeficiency virus-pregnant women in Thailand. Oral Surg Oral Med Oral Pathol Oral Radiol 116(3):306–312. doi:10.1016/j.oooo.2013.04.016
Ramirez V, Gonzalez A, de la Rosa E, Gonzalez M, Rivera I, Hernandez C, Ponce de Leon S (1990) Oral lesions in Mexican HIV-infected patients. J Oral Pathol Med 19(10):482–485
Rautemaa R, Ramage G (2011) Oral candidosis – clinical challenges of a biofilm disease. Crit Rev Microbiol 37(4):328–336. doi:10.3109/1040841X.2011.585606
Recovery.org (2013) Preventing drug and alcohol relapse through self-esteem building for you and your loved ones. http://www.recovery.org/topics/preventing-drug-and-alcohol-relapse-through-self-esteem-building-for-you-and-your-loved-ones/
Santiwongkarn P, Kachonboon S, Thanyasrisung P, Matangkasombut O (2012) Prevalence of oral Candida carriage in Thai adolescents. J Invest Clin Dentist 3(1):51–55. doi:10.1111/j.2041-1626.2011.0089.x
Schulten EA, ten Kate RW, van der Waal I (1989) Oral manifestations of HIV infection in 75 Dutch patients. J Oral Pathol Med 18(1):42–46
Solomon SS, Hawcroft CS, Narasimhan P, Subbaraman R, Srikrishnan AK, Cecelia AJ, Suresh Kumar M, Solomon S, Gallant JE, Celentano DD (2008) Comorbidities among HIV-infected injection drug users in Chennai, India. Indian J Med Res 127(5):447–452
Soysa NS, Ellepola AN (2005) The impact of cigarette/tobacco smoking on oral candidosis: an overview.

Oral Dis 11(5):268–273. doi:10.1111/j.1601-0825.2005.01115.x
Stevens HE (2007) Oral candidiasis secondary to adverse anticholinergic effects of psychotropic medications. J Child Adolesc Psychopharmacol 17(1):145–146. doi:10.1089/cap.2006.0064
Tami-Maury I, Willig J, Vermund S, Jolly P, Aban I, Hill J, Wilson CM (2011) Contemporary profile of oral manifestations of HIV/AIDS and associated risk factors in a Southeastern US clinic. J Public Health Dent 71(4):257–264. doi:10.1111/j.1752-7325.2011.00256.x
Tappuni AR, Fleming GJ (2001) The effect of antiretroviral therapy on the prevalence of oral manifestations in HIV-infected patients: a UK study. Oral Surg Oral Med Oral Pathol Oral Radiol Endod 92(6):623–628. doi:10.1067/moe.2001.118902
Tosello A, Chevaux JM, Montal S, Foti B (2008) Assessment of oral status and oro-pharyngeal candidosis in elderly in short-term hospital care. Odontostomatologie tropicale = Trop Dental J 31(121):43–48
Tukutuku K, Muyembe-Tamfum L, Kayembe K, Odio W, Kandi K, Ntumba M (1990) Oral manifestations of AIDS in a heterosexual population in a Zaire hospital. J Oral Pathol Med 19(5):232–234
Westbrook SD, Kirkpatrick WR, Wiederhold NP, Freytes CO, Toro JJ, Patterson TF, Redding SW (2013) Microbiology and epidemiology of oral yeast colonization in hemopoietic progenitor cell transplant recipients. Oral Surg Oral Med Oral Pathol Oral Radiol 115(3):354–358. doi:10.1016/j.oooo.2012.10.012
Williams DW, Walker R, Lewis MA, Allison RT, Potts AJ (1999) Adherence of Candida albicans to oral epithelial cells differentiated by Papanicolaou staining. J Clin Pathol 52(7):529–531
Wilson MJ, Williams DW, Forbes MD, Finlay IG, Lewis MA (2001) A molecular epidemiological study of sequential oral isolates of Candida albicans from terminally ill patients. J Oral Pathol Med 30(4):206–212
Yan Z, Young AL, Hua H, Xu Y (2011) Multiple oral Candida infections in patients with Sjogren's syndrome – prevalence and clinical and drug susceptibility profiles. J Rheumatol 38(11):2428–2431. doi:10.3899/jrheum.100819
Zhang X, Reichart PA, Song Y (2009) Oral manifestations of HIV/AIDS in China: a review. Oral Maxillofac Surg 13(2):63–68. doi:10.1007/s10006-009-0157-5

Candida Virulence Factors

2

Lindsay E. O'Donnell, Douglas Robertson,
and Gordon Ramage

Abstract

The prevalence of invasive fungal infections has risen significantly worldwide, and although over 600 fungal species are reported as human pathogens, *Candida* species are arguably the most frequently isolated and the most important cause of morbidity and mortality in humans. In fact, *Candida* species are considered the fourth most common cause of hospital-acquired bloodstream infections in the United States. *Candida albicans* is the principal candidal pathogen; however, infections caused by non-*C. albicans* (NCAC) species, such as *C. glabrata, C. dubliniensis, C. tropicalis*, and *C. parapsilosis* have increased considerably. This changing dynamic in NCAC species has been suggested to be due to their intrinsic resistance toward antifungal drugs when compared with *C. albicans*.

Introduction

The prevalence of invasive fungal infections has risen significantly worldwide, and although over 600 fungal species are reported as human pathogens, *Candida* species are arguably the most frequently isolated and the most important cause of morbidity and mortality in humans. In fact, *Candida* species are considered the fourth most common cause of hospital-acquired bloodstream infections in the United States (Lass-Florl 2009). *Candida albicans* is the principal candidal pathogen; however, infections caused by non-*C. albicans* (NCAC) species, such as *C. glabrata, C. dubliniensis, C. tropicalis*, and *C. parapsilosis* have increased considerably. This changing dynamic in NCAC species has been suggested to be due to their intrinsic resistance toward antifungal drugs when compared with *C. albicans* (Silva et al., 2012; Mayer et al., 2013).

Yeasts are part of the microbiota in most individuals and only cause an infection if an opportunity arises. In health, resident yeasts are suppressed by specific and nonspecific defence mechanisms, and also by competitive inhibition from the vast array of other microorganisms (Rodrigues et al., 1999). The increasing occurrence of these infections in recent years has been

L.E. O'Donnell • D. Robertson • G. Ramage (✉)
Glasgow Dental School, School of Medicine,
College of Medical, Veterinary and Life Sciences,
University of Glasgow, Glasgow, UK
e-mail: gordon.ramage@glasgow.ac.uk

E.A.R. Rosa (ed.), *Oral Candidosis: Physiopathology, Decision Making, and Therapeutics*,
DOI 10.1007/978-3-662-47194-4_2

attributed to several factors including the escalated use of immunosuppressive agents, broad-spectrum antibiotics, and implanted medical devices such as catheters and dentures, from which these organisms have the capacity to exist as biofilms, thus adding to their versatility as human pathogens (Ramage et al., 2006). Oropharyngeal candidosis (OPC) is one of the most well-defined candidal infections of humans on soft and hard tissue, forming complex biofilm consortia in association with host components and bacteria (Dongari-Bagtzoglou et al., 2009; Rautemaa and Ramage 2011). Within the context of the wider oral environment, *Candida* species have been shown to be isolated from periodontal pockets, enamel, mucosal surfaces, orthodontic appliances, and dentures (Dongari-Bagtzoglou et al., 2009; Ramage et al., 2004; Sardi et al., 2010; de Carvalho et al., 2006; Arslan et al., 2008). Collectively, various factors influence the onset and severity of OPC, such as the denture material (cleanliness, base material, trauma, duration of wear and its age), smoking and biological factors including cellular immunity, salivary flow, dietary factors, pH of denture plaque, and the oral microbiota composition (Oksala 1990; Coco et al., 2008; Gasparoto et al., 2009).

The success of *Candida* species, and in particular *C. albicans*, as a human pathogenic yeast can almost solely be attributed to their extensive and eloquent arsenal of virulence factors (Fig. 2.1). Arguably, one of the most important and visually striking features of these yeasts relates to phenotypic plasticity, which allows certain members of this genus to adapt to environmental changes through phenotypic switching and the growth of hyphal projections, aiding to their invasion into and through host tissues (Gow et al., 2002). Supplementary to this is the requirement for adhesion to host or biomaterial

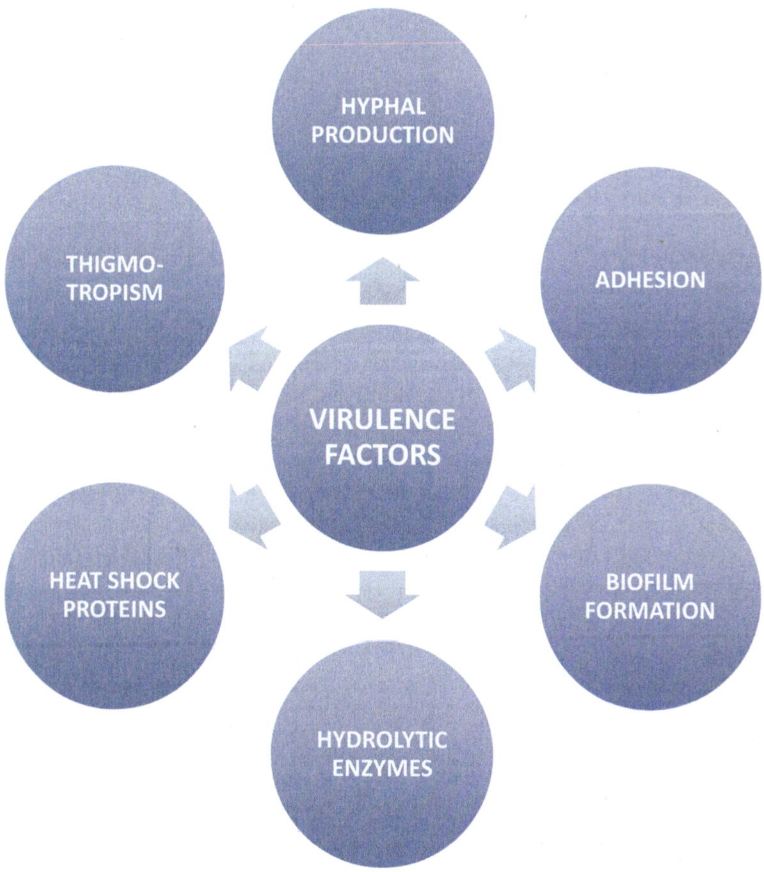

Fig. 2.1 Principal virulence factors assisting in the survival of pathogenic Candida

surfaces, release of hydrolytic enzymes, and protection of cells via the formation of a biofilm. Collectively, these are amongst the principal pathogenic mechanisms assisting in the survival of these pathogenic yeasts (Mayer et al., 2013; Silva et al., 2012).

Adhesion and Colonization

Prior to any signs of overt infection, *Candida* species must first undergo adhesion and colonization to either host cells or an abiotic substrate. After the initial adhesion, colonization is established, which subsequently may lead to a diseased state (Kumamoto 2002). Several factors have been suggested to influence *Candida* adhesion, primarily adhesion proteins (Mayer et al., 2013). The adhesive proteins of *C. albicans* have been intensely studied and the agglutinin-like sequence (ALS) proteins have been identified as the key players. There are eight ALS proteins known, (ALS 1-7 and ALS9) and of these ALS3 has been isolated as the most important due to its vast upregulation during infection and ability to bind cadherins on host cells and induce endocytosis of the pathogen (Murciano et al., 2012; Phan et al., 2007) (Fig. 2.2). Another essential protein is Hwp1, Hyphal-associated GPI-linked protein; this adhesin induces a covalent bond between hyphae and the host cell as Hwp1 is the substrate for transglutaminases. The evidence for the leading role these proteins play comes from studies using knock out (KO) mouse models, which demonstrated reduced infection in models of systemic candidiasis (Sundstrom et al., 2002; Phan et al., 2007). As for *C. albicans* invasive abilities, two invasins are known, Ssa1, a member of the HSP70 family, and the previously mentioned Als3, both bind to E-cadherin on host cells and consequently induce endocytosis (Sun et al., 2010; Phan et al., 2007). *C. glabrata* has lower adherence capacity to gingival cells when compared to *C. albicans* and *C. tropicalis*, and its adhesive properties are under the control of the epithelial adhesion (EPA) family of genes. The *C. glabrata* genome contains several EPA genes, though EPA1 has been shown to play a significant role in adhesion as only EPA1 KO strains have shown reduced adherence (De Las Penas et al., 2003; Cormack et al., 1999). Of note, *C. glabrata* adhere to dentures at a twofold greater rate than *C. albicans*, suggesting that this species have a stronger affinity for binding to prosthetics materials; thus, a possible explanation for the increase in *C. glabrata* infection may simply be due to increased use of denture prosthesis, catheters, and ventilation tubes (Li et al., 2007). In relation to *C. parapsilosis* adhesion during infection, relatively few studies have been undertaken; however, five ALS genes and six predicted glycophosphatidylinositol-anchored proteins 30 (Pga30) have been identified (Butler et al., 2009). As for *C. tropicalis*, it is known to adhere well to human cells and abiotic surfaces and three ALS genes have been recognized thus far. If and how these genes contribute to adhesion is yet to be investigated (Hoyer et al., 2001). Therefore, the knowledge gained from these studies helps to piece together the infection process, giving a better understanding of how subsequent colonization and biofilm formation occurs.

The attachment of fungal cells is closely followed by cell division, proliferation, and the development of a biofilm (Kumamoto 2002). The capacity of some *Candida* species to form biofilms is classed as a virulence factor; a biofilm is defined as a complex structured microbial community enclosed in an extracellular matrix (ECM) and it is now believed that the majority of microorganisms utilize this form of growth. The encased structure of the mature biofilm provides protection by preventing the penetration of host immune factors and antifungals into the ECM when compared to planktonic cells (Ramage et al., 2009). *C. albicans, C. glabrata, C. parapsilosis, and C. tropicalis* all have the ability to form biofilms and have been associated with higher levels of morbidity than that of non-biofilm forming *Candida* species (Kumamoto 2002). Strong evidence suggests the hyphal production of *Candida* species is necessary to form the stable 3D architecture characteristic of mature biofilms (Ganguly and Mitchell 2011). Nonetheless, the need for hyphae to form a biofilm remains controversial as *C. glabrata* is

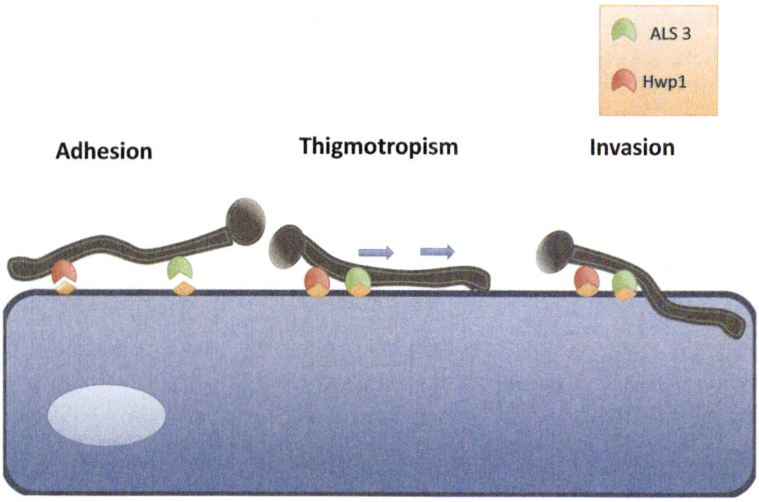

Fig. 2.2 *Key stages in adhesion and tissue penetration. Candida* adheres to epithelial cells via interactions of specific adhesin proteins, such as ALS3 and HWP1, to cellular cadherins. Once adhered, thigmotropism occurs, in which directional hyphal growth leads the hyphae toward weakened areas of the cell. Release of hydrolytic enzymes then further facilitates invasion of the epithelial cell and liberation of nutrients

unable to form hyphae, yet remains the second most commonly isolated *Candida* species (Li et al., 2007). Furthermore, there is a lack of experimental evidence for *C. glabrata* biofilms, despite the increasing number of clinical isolates. Of note, *C. glabrata* is rarely isolated on its own, as it is generally found with other *Candida* species, primarily *C. albicans* (Coco et al., 2008). In cases of severely inflamed denture stomatitis, *C. glabrata* and *C. albicans* were co-isolated in 80 % of cases. Therefore, it has been suggested that the *C. albicans* biofilm supports the growth of *C. glabrata* and acts as a scaffold to maintain structural integrity (El-Azizi et al., 2004; Ramage et al., 2009).

Gene expression is under the control of transcription factors, and these control the upregulation or downregulation of their target genes. Six transcription factors have been identified as the core regulators involved in biofilm formation in *C. albicans*, Egf1, Bcr1, Brg1, Rob1, Ndt80, and Tec1 (Nobile et al., 2012). All of these resulted in defective biofilm formation in vitro and in two in vivo animal models when these genes were deleted (Nobile et al., 2012). The ECM composition of *C. albicans* consists of carbohydrates, mainly β-1,3 glucan, proteins, phosphorus, and hexoamines. Positive regulators of β-1,3 glucan such as Glucoamylases (Gca1 and Gca2), glucan transferases (Bgl2 and Phr1), and exo-glucanase Xog1 play an integral role in protecting the fungal cells as the biofilm becomes more susceptible to antifungals when they are absent (Taff et al., 2012). As for NCAC species, their ECM matrix composition has been understudied; however, it is known that *C. tropicalis* main ECM component is hexosamine and therefore has a lower protein and carbohydrate concentration when compared to other NCAC species (Silva et al., 2009a). Once a mature biofilm is fully established, yeast cells can then disseminate out to other areas, subsequently leading to the spread of infection (Fig. 2.3). Therefore, the formation of a biofilm is a fundamental mechanism exerted by *Candida* species, which aids their success as a pathogen by providing a protective niche for these fungi to grow, proliferate, and subsequently disperse whilst defending against potentially devastating assaults from the immune system.

Although the role of hyphae within biofilms remains controversial, particularly with *C. glabrata*, overwhelming evidence indicates that it plays an integral role of forming the stable 3D architecture.

Filamentation

The genus *Candida* is a group that can grow as several distinct morphologies. The one morphological form in common is the rounded yeast form, although the texture of the colonies differs

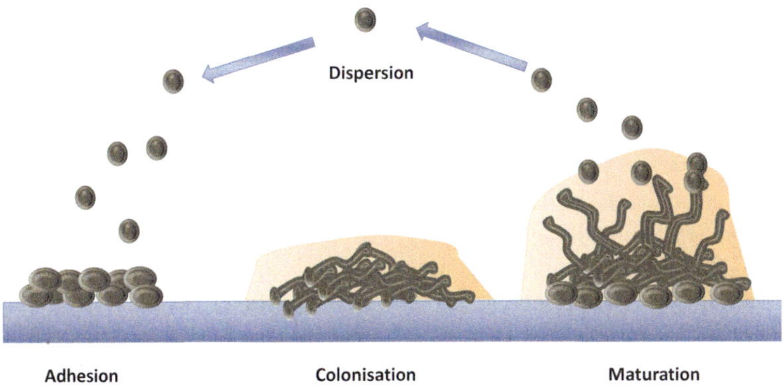

Fig. 2.3 *Developmental phases of biofilm formation*. The attachment of fungal cells is closely followed by cell division and proliferation, thus establishing colonization. The production of hyphal growth and ECM leads to mature stable biofilm architecture. The mature biofilm then disperses yeast cells, subsequently leading to the formation of a new colonies and further biofilm development

depending on the species (Larone 2002b). Hyphae are formed as a germ-tube projection from the original yeast daughter cell, forming branches, which are divided by septa into separate fungal units. Pseudohyphae can also form by budding from the original yeast cell, but which fail to detach and thus extend outward into true hyphae (Silva et al., 2012). Those *Candida* species that can grow as hyphae or pseudohyphae are considered as being more virulent (Jacobsen et al., 2012). This is attributed to its ability to penetrate into mammalian cells more easily than in the yeast form, particularly epithelial cells, which act as a primary barrier for innate immunity. Figure 2.4 illustrates the different morphological forms of *Candida* species.

It is thought that the more effective infiltration of epithelial cells by the filamentous morphologies is due to the pressure generated by the hyphal tip (Gow et al., 2002). The mechanics behind the generation of tip pressure remain little understood; however, it is evident from studies on plant fungal pathogens, that the cell must be sufficiently adhered to the surface to generate the pressure (Brand 2012). This gives explanation as to why genes responsible for adhesion are rapidly upregulated during morphogenesis. The tip is also the site of enzyme secretion and other degrading substances to weaken the cell wall (Hube and Naglik 2001). It has been suggested that the penetrative nature of *Candida* is intrinsic and that these organisms have been programmed to infiltrate any surface they contact. Hyphae are able to penetrate into silicone material that biofilms are grown on, even despite the absence of any biological interactions with the surface (Leonhard et al., 2010). The directionality of hyphal tip growth is responsive to the surrounding environment, allowing the tip to direct its way around obstructions or toward essential nutrients (Gow et al., 1994). Additionally, thigmotropism (directional hyphal growth) can occur due to contact sensing with the cell surface and can lead the hyphae to weakened areas of the cell wall (Hube and Naglik 2001; Gow et al., 1994). Studies on thigmotropism in human pathogenic fungi are limited; however, characteristic thigmotropic behavior has been demonstrated in *C. albicans* and *C. dubliniensis* (Watts et al., 1998; Chen et al., 2011). Control over directionality is important in the initial stages of tissue invasion as a *C. albicans* mutant of the rsr1 gene, which is involved in hyphal directional growth, saw growth become erratic and its invasive abilities decreased by 50 % (Brand et al., 2008). However, once the initial layer of cells has been invaded, control over directional growth is no longer required to cause cell damage (Wachtler et al., 2011). Furthermore, filamentous growth has been suggested as a mechanism for avoiding phagocytosis, with in vitro experiments demonstrating hyphal outgrowth within macrophages leading to puncturing and killing of these cells, though this has yet to be proven in vivo (Cutler 1991).

C. albicans being the most widely studied is known to be truly polymorphic taking on yeast, hyphae, and pseudohyphae forms; this is also true for *C. dubliniensis* (Silva et al., 2012). *C. glabrata* however can only grow as yeast, yet remains to be the second or third most commonly isolated species in candidiasis after *C. albicans*; this is likely a result of the strong antifungal resistance of this species (Li et al., 2007). On the other hand, *C. parapsilosis* fails to generate hyphae but can produce pseudohyphae known as "giant cells" due to their large curved appearance (Trofa et al., 2008). As for *C. tropicalis*, it is found as blastoconidia, pseudohyphae, and may also be found as true hyphae (Larone 2002a; Okawa and Goto 2006). *Candida* morphology is heavily influenced by the environment; for example, pH controls *C. albicans* morphology as pH (<6) grows as yeast and pH (>7) will induce hyphal growth and temperatures of 37 °C and CO_2 also promote filamentous growth (Odds 1988; Sudbery 2011). Quorum sensing, a form of microbial communication, can sense cell densities and which in turn influences cell morphology, the primary quorum sensing molecules in *C. albicans* are farnesol and tyrosol (Albuquerque and Casadevall 2012). As for other NCAC species, there is relatively little evidence on the effect of morphology on the pathogenesis of these species; nonetheless, it is known that *C. tropicalis* can only invade oral epithelium in hyphal formations, only certain strains of *C. parapsilosis* can form hyphae and thus filamentous form was not a requirement to invade oral epithelium (Silva et al., 2009b; Albuquerque and Casadevall 2012; Silva et al., 2011). Perhaps the most prominent evidence for the importance of hyphae as a major virulence factor comes from mutants of *C. albicans* lacking the capacity to form hyphae as they exhibit lower ability to invade cells when compared to wild-type strains (Jayatilake et al., 2006). Thus the combination of hyphal growth, accompanied by thigmotropism, is a successful mechanism of infection. However, invasion is further optimized via the release of hydrolytic enzymes from the hyphal tip, which acts to weaken the cell membrane.

Hydrolytic Enzymes

Damage and penetration of the host epithelium is assisted by the secretion of hydrolytic enzymes in addition to the tip pressure generated by hyphae and pseudohyphae (Wachtler et al., 2012). Several groups of hydrolases are secreted by *Candida* species, proteases, phospholipases, and lipases (Mayer et al., 2013). Secreted aspartyl proteinases (SAP) function by disrupting the host membrane, allowing for pathogenic invasion. Ten SAP proteins have been identified, with some having a more prominent role in pathogenicity than others. SAP1-8 are secreted, whereas SAP9-10 remain bound to the fungal membrane (Naglik et al., 2003; Albrecht et al., 2006). It is well documented that SAP expression is significantly upregulated in *C. albicans* isolates from diseased individuals when compared to healthy controls; furthermore, biofilm formation has also been shown to positively correlate with SAP expression (Naglik et al., 2003). SAP1-3 have been shown to be responsible for the destruction of host epithelium in vitro, (Schaller et al., 1999), whereas SAP5-6 have been linked to hyphal formation and invasive candidal infection, with SAP5 in particular being associated with the early aggressive stage of biofilm formation (Hube et al., 1994; Ramage et al., 2012a). SAP8 is now emerging as a prominent player in candidal infection where it has been shown to be highly upregulated in mature biofilms, yet more evidence is required before a true role for SAP8 can be established (Ramage et al., 2012a). As for the role of SAP in NCAC species, proteinase secretion has been identified in *C. glabrata*, but the class of proteinase was not specified (Chakrabarti et al., 1991). On the other hand, three SAP genes have been identified in *C. parapsilosis*, but they have remained relatively unexplored (Merkerova et al., 2006). *C. parapsilosis* SAP expression appears to be both strain and environment dependant, as it exhibits stronger invasive abilities in skin and vaginal isolates in comparison to strains isolated from oral epithelium (Cassone et al., 1995; Dagdeviren et al., 2005). *C. tropicalis* possesses four SAP genes, named SAPT1-4, with only SAPT1 being well characterized thus far (Zaugg et al., 2001). SAPs secreted from invasive *C. tropicalis* isolates have been found on the fungal cell surface of those penetrating mucosal cells (Borg and Ruchel 1990). However, the role of SAP in invasion remains controversial as recent evidence from a mouse model of oral candidiasis suggests SAP1-6 are not essential causes for infection (Lermann and Morschhauser 2008; Correia et al. 2010). Nonetheless, the vast upregulation of these genes in diseased individuals when compared to healthy indicates they are playing a role in candidal pathogenicity (Hube et al., 1994; Naglik et al., 2008).

Phospholipase production is found in many *Candida* species, *C. albicans* produce several classes, which are separated into four groups, A-D, yet only certain members of class B are secreted extracellularly (PLB1-5), and play a role in virulence (Niewerth and Korting 2001; Mavor et al., 2005). Phospholipases hydrolyze phospholipids into fatty acids and thus cause damage to the host cell membrane and potentially exposing possible adhesion sites (Ghannoum 2000). Evidence for phospholipase secretion in NCAC species has been controversial with some studies reporting phospholipase activity in certain strains, whilst others detected no activity in the same strains (Ghannoum 2000; Kantarcioglu and Yucel 2002). *C. tropicalis* like *C. albicans* exhibits high phospholipase production but it is strain specific (Galan-Ladero et al., 2010; Negri et al., 2010), and as for *C. glabrata*, no studies have been conducted in reference to the presence of phospholipases.

Lipases are involved in the disruption of the cell membrane via the hydrolysis of triacylglycerols (Silva et al., 2012). Ten genes encoding lipases can be found in *C. albicans* LIP1-10, thus far only LIP8 has been proven to have a role in pathogenicity, as a LIP8 mutant showed attenuated virulence in a mouse infection model (Hube et al., 2000; Gacser et al., 2007). *C. parapsilosis* produced a less complicated biofilm when the lipase encoding genes CpLIP1/CpLIP2 were deleted and when a lipase inhibitor was applied; significantly less damage was done to the reconstituted human epithelium (Neugnot et al., 2002). Gene sequences closely related to those in *C. albicans* have been detected in *C. tropicalis*, but not *C. glabrata* (Fu et al., 1997), yet no studies have been conducted to investigate their role in virulence. The evidence for the role of lipases in candidal infection is promising, yet several genes still require exploration before these proteins can be said to be a major virulence factor for *Candida* species.

Stress Response Proteins

Stressful conditions such as starvation within living organisms can induce the heat shock response. Heat shock proteins (HSP) are released to prevent protein unfolding and aggregation, which if not prevented can lead to cell death. They act as chaperones by stabilizing essential proteins, thereby maintaining their form and function (Burnie et al., 2006). To date, six HSPs have been discovered within *C. albicans*: HSP90, HSP60, HSP104, HSP78, and two members of the HSP70 family; Ssa1 and Ssa2 (Mayer et al., 2013). HSP90 is found in all eukaryotes and many of its target protein function as cell-signalling components; however, in *C. albicans*, impaired HSP90 function leads to a temperature-dependant morphological switch from yeast to hyphae (Shapiro et al., 2012). This suggests that HSP90 is having a protective effect by preventing the transition to a more pathogenic morphology. Conversely, compromise of HSP90 induces resistance to azoles and echinocandins, transforming these usually fungistatic class of drugs into fungicidal (Singh et al., 2009; Cowen et al., 2009). Thus, HSP90 has a role in both protection and virulence. However, recent findings in which the depletion of HSP90 in *C. albicans* reduces virulence in a mouse model of systemic fungal infection suggests it is more implicated in pathogenicity (Shapiro et al., 2009). HSP60 is a mitochondrial HSP, of which the function is currently unknown but has been associated with a role in the regulation of elevated temperatures (Leach et al., 2011). As for HSP104 and HSP78, they are involved in biofilm formation and the response to phagocytosis by macrophages, respectively (Lorenz et al., 2004; Fiori et al., 2012). The two HSP70 members

Ssa1 and Ssa2 are expressed on the surface of both yeast and hyphal forms (Li et al., 2006). Mutants of Ssa2 have indicated that this protein is dispensable for virulence; Ssa1 on the other hand acts as an invasin by binding surface proteins and directly infecting the oral epithelium, in a similar fashion as Als3 (Li et al., 2003, Sun et al., 2010).

Additional responses to environmental stress deployed by *C. albicans* include defence against reactive oxygen species (ROS) and reactive nitrogen species (RNS) released by phagocytes. Superoxide dimutases Sod1, Sod5, and catalase Cta1 protect against ROS; meanwhile, flavohemoglobin-related protein Yhb1 defends against RNS; deletion of any of these genes attenuates virulence in mouse models of systemic candidiasis (Brown 2012; Wysong et al., 1998; Hwang et al., 2002; Martchenko et al., 2004; Hromatka et al., 2005).

Antifungal Resistance

The classic treatment for oral candidiasis is antifungal therapy, but finding an effective antifungal is becoming increasingly problematic due to resistance. Resistance develops due to prolonged usage of antifungal drugs, which can have serious consequences, particularly in immunocompromised individuals, and is therefore viewed as an important virulence factor. Resistance can be an innate mechanism but is more commonly acquired by continued exposure to an antifungal where the target organism was previously susceptible.

Several classes of antifungal drugs are currently in use for treatment of candidiasis and are separated into groups depending on their molecular targets. Azoles interfere with membrane component ergosterol, and they target its biosynthesis pathway by inhibiting the enzyme lanosterol demethylase, causing loss of membrane fluidity and function and thus halting cell growth (Lewis et al., 2012). The low toxicity of these agents has led to its overuse in treating fungal infections, which has subsequently resulted in resistance (Pfaller and Diekema 2007). Mutations in the ergosterol biosynthesis pathway as well as the upregulation of efflux pumps are associated with azole resistance (Lupetti et al., 2002; Lewis et al., 2012), with around 20 % of *C. glabrata* strains developing resistance during therapy (Pfaller and Diekema 2007). Fluconazole and itraconozole are active against most *Candida* species with itraconozole showing activity against fluconazole-resistant strains (Pfaller and Diekema 2007; Pfaller et al., 2005). Voriconazole on the other hand acts on most *Candida* species, even those resistant *C. albicans* and *C. glabrata* strains; only *C. tropicalis* is less susceptible (Pfaller and Diekema 2007). Polyenes such as Amphoterecin B (AmpB) are highly fungicidal and directly target the ergosterol membrane components, forming pores, which destabilize the membrane, causing leakage of cellular contents (Lewis et al., 2012). AmpB has the broadest spectrum of antifungal activity and is therefore used to treat chronic fungal infections (Silva et al., 2012). Resistance to polyenes is rare, although in cases that do occur, it is generally a result of mutations in key members of the ergosterol biosynthesis pathway, which reduce the amount of ergosterol in the membrane. Mutations of enzyme sterol delta 5,6-denaturase (ERG3), which contribute to lowering antifungal susceptibility, are thought to be the primary cause (Chau et al., 2005). The most recent addition to the antifungal family are echinocandins, and these agents work by inhibiting β-1,3-D-glucan synthase, an enzyme essential for the synthesis of the key cell wall component β-1,3-D-glucan (Fig. 2.4) (Denning 2003). The echinocandins are active against *C. albicans, C. glabrata, C. tropicalis* but higher MIC values are required against *C. parapsilosis* (Pfaller et al., 2005). As this group of agents are relatively new, their use has not been widespread enough to determine if resistance against these antifungals will arise.

However, subinhibitory concentrations of these drugs are sufficient to induce an immune response by exposing β-glucans normally buried beneath mannoproteins on the cell membrane surface; it has been suggested that this may even occur in echinocandin-resistant strains and thus may be a limiting factor for the emergence of resistance during treatment (Wheeler and Fink 2006; Ben-Ami and Kontoyiannis 2012; Ben-Ami et al., 2011).

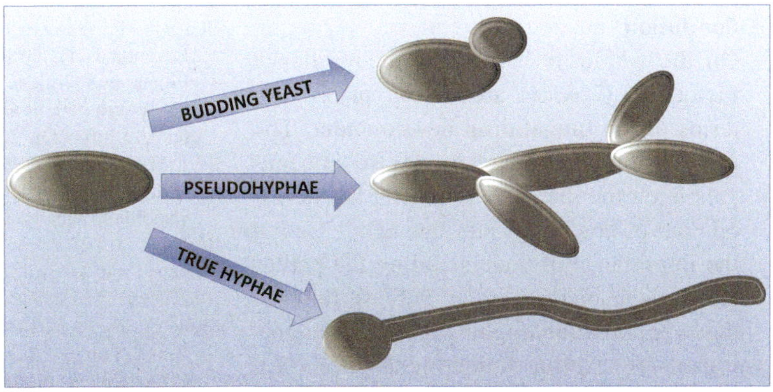

Fig. 2.4 *The different morphological forms of Candida.* This schematic diagram provides a pictorial representation of the key forms of cells associated with *Candida albicans*

Reduced susceptibility to antifungal agents can be largely attributed to the biofilm and its resistance mechanisms. For example cells within a biofilm have been found to be more resistant than planktonic cells and the denser the biofilm network is the less susceptible the cells within become (Douglas 2003). In addition, the components of the extracellular matrix (ECM) are thought to greatly contribute to resistance (Ramage et al., 2012b). Extracellular DNA is found within the ECM of *C. albicans* and its depletion using DNAse increases susceptibility to polyenes and echinocandins (Ramage et al., 2012b; Martins et al., 2012). Furthermore, the cell wall constituent β-1,3-D-glucan is the primary carbohydrate found in the ECM and investigations have shown that this molecule sequesters antifungals including azoles, polyenes, and echinocandins by acting as a "sponge" within *C. albicans* biofilms (Nett et al., 2010a, b).

Moreover, it has been suggested that the increase in efflux pumps is the primary factor responsible for resistance. These pumps are controlled by the ATP-binding cassette (ABC) consisting of a membrane pore with two ABC pumps providing the energy source (Albertson et al., 1996; Lopez-Ribot et al., 1999). The CDR family of genes associated with this mechanism are upregulated during biofilm formation; however, studies have shown their role in conferring resistance occurs during the early stages but less so once the biofilm has matured as *C. albicans* strains deficient in efflux pumps are extremely susceptible to fluconazole at 6 h but become highly resistant at 12 and 48 h (Mukherjee et al., 2003). *C. glabrata* has also shown similar patterns of increased CDR gene expression during biofilm formation, several gain of function mutations have been identified within these genes in *C. glabrata*, which may explain its increased resistance compared to other *Candida* species (Li et al. 2007), whilst *C. tropicalis* demonstrates upregulation of the secondary transporter MDR. Thus, efflux pumps, whilst playing an important role, are not exclusive in causing resistance.

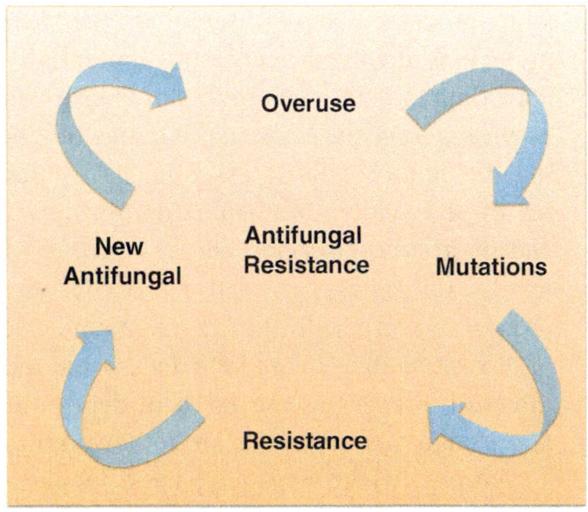

Fig. 2.5 Vicious development of resistance to new antifungals

The problem of resistance currently is being treated with the introduction of new antifungals to treat infections; however, these new agents soon follow the same pattern as their predecessors, being overused, which subsequently leads to resistance (Fig. 2.5). Therefore, more research is required to find an effective treatment, which simultaneously blocks resistance mechanisms whilst treating the fungal infection.

Conclusion

On the whole, research into the virulence factors of *Candida* are of top priority in terms of antifungal drug development. The progression of drug resistance to antifungals is on the increase, requiring the development of new drugs and thus emphasizing the importance of understanding the pathogenic mechanisms exerted by these fungi to uncover potential drug targets. These microorganisms exhibit unique characteristics, which optimize their success as a pathogen; in depth studies on the adhesion and invasion processes have identified the key molecules involved, suggesting potentially appealing targets. The process of invasion is now relatively well understood, and blocking the action of those essential molecules involved in polymorphism, thigmotropism and hydrolytic enzymes, the key processes involved in invasion, will likely become prospective targets for future treatments. All of this research is key to help understand the infection process as the more in depth our knowledge, the closer we are to developing a treatment where resistance is no longer a problem.

References

Albertson GD, Niimi M, Cannon RD, Jenkinson HF (1996) Multiple efflux mechanisms are involved in Candida albicans fluconazole resistance. Antimicrob Agents Chemother 40:2835–2841

Albrecht A, Felk A, Pichova I, Naglik JR, Schaller M, De Groot P, Maccallum D, Odds FC, Schafer W, Klis F, Monod M, Hube B (2006) Glycosylphosphatidylinositol-anchored proteases of Candida albicans target proteins necessary for both cellular processes and host-pathogen interactions. J Biol Chem 281:688–694

Albuquerque P, Casadevall A (2012) Quorum sensing in fungi – a review. Med Mycol 50:337–345

Arslan SG, Akpolat N, Kama JD, Ozer T, Hamamci O (2008) One-year follow-up of the effect of fixed orthodontic treatment on colonization by oral Candida. J Oral Pathol Med 37:26–29

Ben-Ami R, Kontoyiannis DP (2012) Resistance to echinocandins comes at a cost. The impact of FKS1 hotspot mutations on Candida albicans fitness and virulence. Virulence 3:95–97

Ben-Ami R, Garcia-Effron G, Lewis RE, Gamarra S, Leventakos K, Perlin DS, Kontoyiannis DP (2011) Fitness and virulence costs of Candida albicans FKS1 hot spot mutations associated with echinocandin resistance. J Infect Dis 204:626–635

Borg M, Ruchel R (1990) Demonstration of fungal proteinase during phagocytosis of Candida albicans and Candida tropicalis. J Med Vet Mycol 28:3–14

Brand A (2012) Hyphal growth in human fungal pathogens and its role in virulence. Int J Microbiol 2012:517529

Brand A, Vacharaksa A, Bendel C, Norton J, Haynes P, Henry-Stanley M, Wells C, Ross K, Gow NA, Gale CA (2008) An internal polarity landmark is important for externally induced hyphal behaviors in Candida albicans. Eukaryot Cell 7:712–720

Brown AJ (2012) Stress responses in Candida. *Candida and Candidiasis*. ASM Press, Washington, DC

Burnie JP, Carter TL, Hodgetts SJ, Matthews RC (2006) Fungal heat-shock proteins in human disease. FEMS Microbiol Rev 30:53–88

Butler G, Rasmussen MD, Lin MF, Santos MA, Sakthikumar S, Munro CA, Rheinbay E, Grabherr M, Forche A, Reedy JL, Agrafioti I, Arnaud MB, Bates S, Brown AJ, Brunke S, Costanzo MC, Fitzpatrick DA, De Groot PW, Harris D, Hoyer LL, Hube B, Klis FM, Kodira C, Lennard N, Logue ME, Martin R, Neiman AM, Nikolaou E, Quail MA, Quinn J, Santos MC, Schmitzberger FF, Sherlock G, Shah P, Silverstein KA, Skrzypek MS, Soll D, Staggs R, Stansfield I, Stumpf MP, Sudbery PE, Srikantha T, Zeng Q, Berman J, Berriman M, Heitman J, Gow NA, Lorenz MC, Birren BW, Kellis M, Cuomo CA (2009) Evolution of pathogenicity and sexual reproduction in eight Candida genomes. Nature 459:657–662

Cassone A, De Bernardis F, Pontieri E, Carruba G, Girmenia C, Martino P, Fernandez-Rodriguez M, Quindos G, Ponton J (1995) Biotype diversity of Candida parapsilosis and its relationship to the clinical source and experimental pathogenicity. J Infect Dis 171:967–975

Chakrabarti A, Nayak N, Talwar P (1991) In vitro proteinase production by Candida species. Mycopathologia 114:163–168

Chau AS, Gurnani M, Hawkinson R, Laverdiere M, Cacciapuoti A, Mcnicholas PM (2005) Inactivation of sterol Delta 5,6-desaturase attenuates virulence in Candida albicans. Antimicrob Agents Chemother 49:3646–3651

Chen YL, Brand A, Morrison EL, Silao FG, Bigol UG, Malbas FF Jr, Nett JE, Andes DR, Solis NV, Filler SG, Averette A, Heitman J (2011) Calcineurin controls drug tolerance, hyphal growth, and virulence in Candida dubliniensis. Eukaryot Cell 10:803–819

Coco BJ, Bagg J, Cross LJ, Jose A, Cross J, Ramage G (2008) Mixed Candida albicans and Candida glabrata populations associated with the pathogenesis of denture stomatitis. Oral Microbiol Immunol 23: 377–383

Cormack BP, Ghori N, Falkow S (1999) An adhesin of the yeast pathogen Candida glabrata mediating adherence to human epithelial cells. Science 285:578–582

Correia A, Lermann U, Teixeira L, Cerca F, Botelho S, Da Costa RM, Sampaio P, Gartner F, Morschhauser J, Vilanova M, Pais C (2010) Limited role of secreted aspartyl proteinases Sap1 to Sap6 in Candida albicans virulence and host immune response in murine hematogenously disseminated candidiasis. Infect Immun 78:4839–4849

Cowen LE, Singh SD, Kohler JR, Collins C, Zaas AK, Schell WA, Aziz H, Mylonakis E, Perfect JR, Whitesell L, Lindquist S (2009) Harnessing Hsp90 function as a powerful, broadly effective therapeutic strategy for fungal infectious disease. Proc Natl Acad Sci U S A 106:2818–2823

Cutler JE (1991) Putative virulence factors of Candida albicans. Annu Rev Microbiol 45:187–218

Dagdeviren M, Cerikcioglu N, Karavus M (2005) Acid proteinase, phospholipase and adherence properties of Candida parapsilosis strains isolated from clinical specimens of hospitalised patients. Mycoses 48:321–326

De Carvalho FG, Silva DS, Hebling J, Spolidorio LC, Spolidorio DM (2006) Presence of mutans streptococci and Candida spp. in dental plaque/dentine of carious teeth and early childhood caries. Arch Oral Biol 51:1024–1028

De Las Penas A, Pan SJ, Castano I, Alder J, Cregg R, Cormack BP (2003) Virulence-related surface glycoproteins in the yeast pathogen Candida glabrata are encoded in subtelomeric clusters and subject to RAP1- and SIR-dependent transcriptional silencing. Genes Dev 17:2245–2258

Denning DW (2003) Echinocandin antifungal drugs. Lancet 362:1142–1151

Dongari-Bagtzoglou A, Kashleva H, Dwivedi P, Diaz P, Vasilakos J (2009) Characterization of mucosal Candida albicans biofilms. PLoS One 4, e7967

Douglas LJ (2003) Candida biofilms and their role in infection. Trends Microbiol 11:30–36

El-Azizi MA, Starks SE, Khardori N (2004) Interactions of Candida albicans with other Candida spp. and bacteria in the biofilms. J Appl Microbiol 96:1067–1073

Fiori A, Kucharikova S, Govaert G, Cammue BP, Thevissen K, Van Dijck P (2012) The heat-induced molecular disaggregase Hsp104 of Candida albicans plays a role in biofilm formation and pathogenicity in a worm infection model. Eukaryot Cell 11:1012–1020

Fu Y, Ibrahim AS, Fonzi W, Zhou X, Ramos CF, Ghannoum MA (1997) Cloning and characterization of a gene (LIP1) which encodes a lipase from the pathogenic yeast Candida albicans. Microbiology-UK 143:331–340

Gacser A, Trofa D, Schafer W, Nosanchuk JD (2007) Targeted gene deletion in Candida parapsilosis demonstrates the role of secreted lipase in virulence. J Clin Invest 117:3049–3058

Galan-Ladero MA, Blanco MT, Sacristan B, Fernandez-Calderon MC, Perez-Giraldo C, Gomez-Garcia AC (2010) Enzymatic activities of Candida tropicalis isolated from hospitalized patients. Med Mycol 48:207–210

Ganguly S, Mitchell AP (2011) Mucosal biofilms of Candida albicans. Curr Opin Microbiol 14:380–385

Gasparoto TH, Vieira NA, Porto VC, Campanelli AP, Lara VS (2009) Ageing exacerbates damage of systemic and salivary neutrophils from patients presenting Candida-related denture stomatitis. Immun Ageing 6:3

Ghannoum MA (2000) Potential role of phospholipases in virulence and fungal pathogenesis. Clin Microbiol Rev 13:122–143, Table of contents

Gow NA, Perera TH, Sherwood-Higham J, Gooday GW, Gregory DW, Marshall D (1994) Investigation of touch-sensitive responses by hyphae of the human pathogenic fungus Candida albicans. Scanning Microsc 8:705–710

Gow NA, Brown AJ, Odds FC (2002) Fungal morphogenesis and host invasion. Curr Opin Microbiol 5:366–371

Hoyer LL, Fundyga R, Hecht JE, Kapteyn JC, Klis FM, Arnold J (2001) Characterization of agglutinin-like sequence genes from non-albicans Candida and phylogenetic analysis of the ALS family. Genetics 157:1555–1567

Hromatka BS, Noble SM, Johnson AD (2005) Transcriptional response of Candida albicans to nitric oxide and the role of the YHB1 gene in nitrosative stress and virulence. Mol Biol Cell 16:4814–4826

Hube B, Naglik J (2001) Candida albicans proteinases: resolving the mystery of a gene family. Microbiology 147:1997–2005

Hube B, Monod M, Schofield DA, Brown AJ, Gow NA (1994) Expression of seven members of the gene family encoding secretory aspartyl proteinases in Candida albicans. Mol Microbiol 14:87–99

Hube B, Stehr F, Bossenz M, Mazur A, Kretschmar M, Schafer W (2000) Secreted lipases of Candida albicans: cloning, characterisation and expression analysis of a new gene family with at least ten members. Arch Microbiol 174:362–374

Hwang CS, Rhie GE, Oh JH, Huh WK, Yim HS, Kang SO (2002) Copper- and zinc-containing superoxide dismutase (Cu/ZnSOD) is required for the protection of Candida albicans against oxidative stresses and the expression of its full virulence. Microbiology 148:3705–3713

Jacobsen ID, Wilson D, Wachtler B, Brunke S, Naglik JR, Hube B (2012) Candida albicans dimorphism as a therapeutic target. Expert Rev Anti Infect Ther 10:85–93

Jayatilake JA, Samaranayake YH, Cheung LK, Samaranayake LP (2006) Quantitative evaluation of tissue invasion by wild type, hyphal and SAP mutants of Candida albicans, and non-albicans Candida species in reconstituted human oral epithelium. J Oral Pathol Med 35:484–491

Kantarcioglu AS, Yucel A (2002) Phospholipase and protease activities in clinical Candida isolates with reference to the sources of strains. Mycoses 45:160–165

Kumamoto CA (2002) Candida biofilms. Curr Opin Microbiol 5:608–611

Larone D (2002a) Medically important fungi; a guide to identification. ASM Press, Washington, DC
Larone D (2002b) Medically important fungi: a guide to identification. ASM Press, Washington, DC
Lass-Florl C (2009) The changing face of epidemiology of invasive fungal disease in Europe. Mycoses 52:197–205
Leach MD, Stead DA, Argo E, Brown AJ (2011) Identification of sumoylation targets, combined with inactivation of SMT3, reveals the impact of sumoylation upon growth, morphology, and stress resistance in the pathogen Candida albicans. Mol Biol Cell 22:687–702
Leonhard M, Moser D, Reumueller A, Mancusi G, Bigenzahn W, Schneider-Stickler B (2010) Comparison of biofilm formation on new Phonax and Provox 2 voice prostheses - a pilot study. Head Neck 32:886–895
Lermann U, Morschhauser J (2008) Secreted aspartic proteases are not required for invasion of reconstituted human epithelia by Candida albicans. Microbiology 154:3281–3295
Lewis RE, Viale P, Kontoyiannis DP (2012) The potential impact of antifungal drug resistance mechanisms on the host immune response to Candida. Virulence 3:368–376
Li XS, Reddy MS, Baev D, Edgerton M (2003) Candida albicans Ssa1/2p is the cell envelope binding protein for human salivary histatin 5. J Biol Chem 278:28553–28561
Li XS, Sun JN, Okamoto-Shibayama K, Edgerton M (2006) Candida albicans cell wall ssa proteins bind and facilitate import of salivary histatin 5 required for toxicity. J Biol Chem 281:22453–22463
Li L, Redding S, Dongari-Bagtzoglou A (2007) Candida glabrata: an emerging oral opportunistic pathogen. J Dent Res 86:204–215
Lopez-Ribot JL, Mcatee RK, Perea S, Kirkpatrick WR, Rinaldi MG, Patterson TF (1999) Multiple resistant phenotypes of Candida albicans coexist during episodes of oropharyngeal candidiasis in human immunodeficiency virus-infected patients. Antimicrob Agents Chemother 43:1621–1630
Lorenz MC, Bender JA, Fink GR (2004) Transcriptional response of Candida albicans upon internalization by macrophages. Eukaryot Cell 3:1076–1087
Lupetti A, Danesi R, Campa M, Del Tacca M, Kelly S (2002) Molecular basis of resistance to azole antifungals. Trends Mol Med 8:76–81
Martchenko M, Alarco AM, Harcus D, Whiteway M (2004) Superoxide dismutases in Candida albicans: transcriptional regulation and functional characterization of the hyphal-induced SOD5 gene. Mol Biol Cell 15:456–467
Martins M, Henriques M, Lopez-Ribot JL, Oliveira R (2012) Addition of DNase improves the in vitro activity of antifungal drugs against Candida albicans biofilms. Mycoses 55:80–85
Mavor AL, Thewes S, Hube B (2005) Systemic fungal infections caused by Candida species: epidemiology, infection process and virulence attributes. Curr Drug Targets 6:863–874
Mayer FL, Wilson D, Hube B (2013) Candida albicans pathogenicity mechanisms. Virulence 4:119–128
Merkerova M, Dostal J, Hradilek M, Pichova I, Hruskova-Heidingsfeldova O (2006) Cloning and characterization of Sapp2p, the second aspartic proteinase isoenzyme from Candida parapsilosis. FEMS Yeast Res 6:1018–1026
Mukherjee PK, Chandra J, Kuhn DM, Ghannoum MA (2003) Mechanism of fluconazole resistance in Candida albicans biofilms: phase-specific role of efflux pumps and membrane sterols. Infect Immun 71:4333–4340
Murciano C, Moyes DL, Runglall M, Tobouti P, Islam A, Hoyer LL, Naglik JR (2012) Evaluation of the role of Candida albicans agglutinin-like sequence (Als) proteins in human oral epithelial cell interactions. PLoS One 7, e33362
Naglik JR, Challacombe SJ, Hube B (2003) Candida albicans secreted aspartyl proteinases in virulence and pathogenesis. Microbiol Mol Biol Rev 67:400–428, Table of contents
Naglik JR, Moyes D, Makwana J, Kanzaria P, Tsichlaki E, Weindl G, Tappuni AR, Rodgers CA, Woodman AJ, Challacombe SJ, Schaller M, Hube B (2008) Quantitative expression of the Candida albicans secreted aspartyl proteinase gene family in human oral and vaginal candidiasis. Microbiology 154:3266–3280
Negri M, Martins M, Henriques M, Svidzinski TI, Azeredo J, Oliveira R (2010) Examination of potential virulence factors of Candida tropicalis clinical isolates from hospitalized patients. Mycopathologia 169:175–182
Nett JE, Crawford K, Marchillo K, Andes DR (2010a) Role of Fks1p and matrix glucan in Candida albicans biofilm resistance to an echinocandin, pyrimidine, and polyene. Antimicrob Agents Chemother 54:3505–3508
Nett JE, Sanchez H, Cain MT, Andes DR (2010b) Genetic basis of Candida biofilm resistance due to drug-sequestering matrix glucan. J Infect Dis 202:171–175
Neugnot V, Moulin G, Dubreucq E, Bigey F (2002) The lipase/acyltransferase from Candida parapsilosis: molecular cloning and characterization of purified recombinant enzymes. Eur J Biochem 269:1734–1745
Niewerth M, Korting HC (2001) Phospholipases of Candida albicans. Mycoses 44:361–367
Nobile CJ, Fox EP, Nett JE, Sorrells TR, Mitrovich QM, Hernday AD, Tuch BB, Andes DR, Johnson AD (2012) A recently evolved transcriptional network controls biofilm development in Candida albicans. Cell 148:126–138
Odds FC (1988) Candida and Candidosis. Bailliere Tindall, London
Okawa Y, Goto K (2006) Antigenicity of Candida tropicalis strain cells cultured at 27 and 37 degrees C. FEMS Immunol Med Microbiol 46:438–443
Oksala E (1990) Factors predisposing to oral yeast infections. Acta Odontol Scand 48:71–74
Pfaller MA, Diekema DJ (2007) Epidemiology of invasive candidiasis: a persistent public health problem. Clin Microbiol Rev 20:133–163
Pfaller MA, Boyken L, Hollis RJ, Messer SA, Tendolkar S, Diekema DJ (2005) In vitro susceptibilities of clinical isolates of Candida species, Cryptococcus neoformans, and Aspergillus species to itraconazole: global

survey of 9,359 isolates tested by clinical and laboratory standards institute broth microdilution methods. J Clin Microbiol 43:3807–3810
Phan QT, Myers CL, Fu Y, Sheppard DC, Yeaman MR, Welch WH, Ibrahim AS, Edwards JE, Filler SG (2007) Als3 is a Candida albicans invasin that binds to cadherins and induces endocytosis by host cells. Plos Biol 5:543–557
Ramage G, Tomsett K, Wickes BL, Lopez-Ribot JL, Redding SW (2004) Denture stomatitis: a role for Candida biofilms. Oral Surg Oral Med Oral Pathol Oral Radiol Endod 98:53–59
Ramage G, Martinez JP, Lopez-Ribot JL (2006) Candida biofilms on implanted biomaterials: a clinically significant problem. FEMS Yeast Res 6:979–986
Ramage G, Mowat E, Jones B, Williams C, Lopez-Ribot J (2009) Our current understanding of fungal biofilms. Crit Rev Microbiol 35:340–355
Ramage G, Coco B, Sherry L, Bagg J, Lappin DF (2012a) In vitro Candida albicans biofilm induced proteinase activity and SAP8 expression correlates with in vivo denture stomatitis severity. Mycopathologia 174:11–19
Ramage G, Rajendran R, Sherry L, Williams C (2012b) Fungal biofilm resistance. Int J Microbiol 2012:528521
Rautemaa R, Ramage G (2011) Oral candidosis – clinical challenges of a biofilm disease. Crit Rev Microbiol 37:328–336
Rodrigues AG, Mardh PA, Pina-Vaz C, Martinez-De-Oliveira J, Da Fonseca AF (1999) Is the lack of concurrence of bacterial vaginosis and vaginal candidosis explained by the presence of bacterial amines? Am J Obstet Gynecol 181:367–370
Sardi JC, Duque C, Mariano FS, Peixoto IT, Hofling JF, Goncalves RB (2010) Candida spp. in periodontal disease: a brief review. J Oral Sci 52:177–185
Schaller M, Korting HC, Schafer W, Bastert J, Chen W, Hube B (1999) Secreted aspartic proteinase (Sap) activity contributes to tissue damage in a model of human oral candidosis. Mol Microbiol 34:169–180
Shapiro RS, Uppuluri P, Zaas AK, Collins C, Senn H, Perfect JR, Heitman J, Cowen LE (2009) Hsp90 orchestrates temperature-dependent Candida albicans morphogenesis via Ras1-PKA signaling. Curr Biol 19:621–629
Shapiro RS, Zaas AK, Betancourt-Quiroz M, Perfect JR, Cowen LE (2012) The Hsp90 co-chaperone Sgt1 governs Candida albicans morphogenesis and drug resistance. PLoS One 7, e44734
Silva S, Henriques M, Martins A, Oliveira R, Williams D, Azeredo J (2009a) Biofilms of non-Candida albicans Candida species: quantification, structure and matrix composition. Med Mycol 47:681–689
Silva S, Henriques M, Oliveira R, Azeredo J, Malic S, Hooper SJ, Williams DW (2009b) Characterization of Candida parapsilosis infection of an in vitro reconstituted human oral epithelium. Eur J Oral Sci 117:669–675
Silva S, Hooper SJ, Henriques M, Oliveira R, Azeredo J, Williams DW (2011) The role of secreted aspartyl proteinases in Candida tropicalis invasion and damage of oral mucosa. Clin Microbiol Infect 17:264–272
Silva S, Negri M, Henriques M, Oliveira R, Williams DW, Azeredo J (2012) Candida glabrata, Candida parapsilosis and Candida tropicalis: biology, epidemiology, pathogenicity and antifungal resistance. FEMS Microbiol Rev 36:288–305
Singh SD, Robbins N, Zaas AK, Schell WA, Perfect JR, Cowen LE (2009) Hsp90 governs echinocandin resistance in the pathogenic yeast Candida albicans via calcineurin. PLoS Pathog 5, e1000532
Sudbery PE (2011) Growth of Candida albicans hyphae. Nat Rev Microbiol 9:737–748
Sun JN, Solis NV, Phan QT, Bajwa JS, Kashleva H, Thompson A, Liu Y, Dongari-Bagtzoglou A, Edgerton M, Filler SG (2010) Host cell invasion and virulence mediated by Candida albicans Ssa1. PLoS Pathog 6, e1001181
Sundstrom P, Balish E, Allen CM (2002) Essential role of the Candida albicans transglutaminase substrate, hyphal wall protein 1, in lethal oroesophageal candidiasis in immunodeficient mice. J Infect Dis 185:521–530
Taff HT, Nett JE, Zarnowski R, Ross KM, Sanchez H, Cain MT, Hamaker J, Mitchell AP, Andes DR (2012) A Candida biofilm-induced pathway for matrix glucan delivery: implications for drug resistance. PLoS Pathog 8, e1002848
Trofa D, Gacser A, Nosanchuk JD (2008) Candida parapsilosis, an emerging fungal pathogen. Clin Microbiol Rev 21:606–625
Wachtler B, Wilson D, Haedicke K, Dalle F, Hube B (2011) From attachment to damage: defined genes of Candida albicans mediate adhesion, invasion and damage during interaction with oral epithelial cells. PLoS One 6, e17046
Wachtler B, Citiulo F, Jablonowski N, Forster S, Dalle F, Schaller M, Wilson D, Hube B (2012) Candida albicans-epithelial interactions: dissecting the roles of active penetration, induced endocytosis and host factors on the infection process. PLoS One 7, e36952
Watts HJ, Very AA, Perera TH, Davies JM, Gow NA (1998) Thigmotropism and stretch-activated channels in the pathogenic fungus Candida albicans. Microbiology 144(Pt 3):689–695
Wheeler RT, Fink GR (2006) A drug-sensitive genetic network masks fungi from the immune system. PLoS Pathog 2, e35
Wysong DR, Christin L, Sugar AM, Robbins PW, Diamond RD (1998) Cloning and sequencing of a Candida albicans catalase gene and effects of disruption of this gene. Infect Immun 66:1953–1961
Zaugg C, Borg-Von Zepelin M, Reichard U, Sanglard D, Monod M (2001) Secreted aspartic proteinase family of Candida tropicalis. Infect Immun 69:405–412

Immunological Features Protect Against *Candida* spp.

3

Denise M. Palomari Spolidorio,
Renata Serignoli Francisconi,
Luís Carlos Spolidorio,
and Edvaldo Antonio Ribeiro Rosa

Abstract

The epithelial mucosa is an important component of the host immune defense and immune surveillance since it is the first layer that most microorganisms initially contact. The most important function of the immune system is to discriminate between self and nonself, a property that is essential for the maintenance of immune homeostasis. This specialized interaction results in passive coexistence of microorganisms with host, as in the case of commensal microorganisms, or a breach of the mucosa barrier and subsequent cell injury, as occurs during infection with microbial pathogens.

The epithelial mucosa is an important component of the host immune defense and immune surveillance since it is the first layer that most microorganisms initially contact. The most important function of the immune system is to discriminate between self and nonself, a property that is essential for the maintenance of immune homeostasis. This specialized interaction results in passive coexistence of microorganisms with host, as in the case of commensal microorganisms, or a breach of the mucosal barrier and subsequent cell injury, as occurs in during infection with microbial pathogens.

Fungal infections, also known as mycosis if they are caused by *Candida*, often start at mucosal surfaces and the innate immune response is responsible for preventing the spread of the microorganisms (Maródi et al., 1991). The cells that compose the innate immune response are

D.M.P. Spolidorio (✉)
Department of Physiology and Pathology, Araraquara Dental School, State University of São Paulo, São Paulo, Brazil
e-mail: dmps@foar.unesp.br

R.S. Francisconi
Department of Physiology and Pathology, Araraquara Dental School, State University of São Paulo, São Paulo, Brazil

L.C. Spolidorio
Department of Physiology and Pathology, Araraquara School of Dentistry, Sao Paulo State University (UNESP), Araraquara, SP, Brazil

E.A.R. Rosa
School of Health and Biosciences, Xenobiotics Research Unit, The Pontifical Catholic University of Paraná, Curitiba, Brazil

E.A.R. Rosa (ed.), *Oral Candidosis: Physiopathology, Decision Making, and Therapeutics*,
DOI 10.1007/978-3-662-47194-4_3

phagocytes, including neutrophils and macrophages, which perform phagocytosis, and dendritic cells and natural killer (NK) cells. Additionally, the innate immune system consists of physical barriers, such as epithelia, and chemical barriers, including antimicrobial substances produced by epithelial cells, cytokines, and complement system proteins that are produced by various cell types and that regulate the activity of cells of innate immunity.

The barrier function alone is usually sufficient to contain commensal organisms, but is often insufficient to protect against pathogenic microorganisms. However, research has revealed that skin cells are able to trigger an immune response similar to myeloid lineage cells and, therefore, play an important role in the recognition of active microorganisms. Thus, the oral epithelium is able to secrete a variety of effector molecules that defend against infectious agents and mediate an inflammatory immune response by activating myeloid cells in the submucosal layers in order to get rid of invading pathogens.

The incidence of fungal infections in the skin and mucous membranes is increasing worldwide due to multiple predisposing factors, which facilitate the conversion of commensal parasites existences, and the increase in infections associated with immune deficiencies. *Candida albicans* and related species are found ubiquitously and are commensal microbiota in the rectal, oral, vaginal, urethral, nasal and cavities, and on human skin. It is considered the gateway to opportunistic pathogens, leading to the risk of systemic dissemination in immunocompromised individuals (Dillon et al., 2006; Fidel et al., 1997). This group is not only composed of patients with primary or acquired immunodeficiency, but also those with conditions that are paradoxically linked to the advancement of medicine and surgery, such as admissions to ICUs, organ transplantation, use of broad-spectrum antibiotics, and chemotherapy (Eggimann et al., 2011). Immunodeficiency is a complicating factor for clinically relevant infections because neutrophil deficiency is often associated with such infections.

The host–fungus interaction presents a dynamic feature that needs to be taken into consideration. The fungi can quickly change into different morphological forms (dimorphism), and this property can have profound implications on the outcome of an infection. *C. albicans* can be detected in different forms, such as yeast, pseudohyphae, and hyphae chlamydospores, and each has been isolated clinically and has a specific pattern of genes expression. While the spread of yeast secured *C. albicans* hyphae facilitates the tissue invasion or biofilm formation, chlamydospores are responsible for allowing survival in hostile environments. Both surface and invasive fungal infections can develop if there is a change in location of either the immune system of the patient or the microbiota (Eggimann et al., 2011). An important clinical relevance of *Candida* is its ability to form biofilms on surfaces, resulting in changes in immunity, either local or systemic, which can lead to disease development (Miceli et al., 2011).

C. albicans is able to induce various morphological changes, such as the transition from yeast to hyphae in response to various stimuli of the host (e.g., CO_2 or serum). This complicates the dynamic phenotype characterization of the host immune response against *C. albicans*. In particular, during the transition into morphogenetic *C. albicans* masks some cell wall components and debunks others, qualitatively changing the presentation of certain PAMPs to the host.

Virulence factors are crucial in determining the role of opportunistic pathogens during infections. In addition to dimorphism, other virulence factors expressed by *Candida* include adhesion factors, phenotypic switching, thigmotropism (ability to identify intercellular junctions in the mucosal surface for penetration), and secretion of hydrolytic enzymes, such as lipase, phospholipase, and proteinase.

Compared to bacterial infections, fungal infections have added complications when it comes to control or prevention of disease due to the limited number of antifungal agents. Moreover, diagnosis is difficult by conventional culture methods. An ideal antifungal agent should have low resistance and minimal drug interactions, as well as a wide range and flexibility for application (Chapman et al., 2008). Currently on the market, there are three classes of natural products (griseofulvin, polyenes, and echinocandins) and four classes of synthetic chemicals (allylamines, azoles, flucytosine, and phenylmorpholine) with clinical value against fungi. Due to the large amount of morbidity and mortality caused by fungal infections, the use of these drugs is considered a better alternative to trying to control the infections (Odds 2003).

Immune Responses Specific to Fungi

Candidiasis: Gastrointestinal (GI) Tract

The primary protective responses to fungal infection are promoted by pro-inflammatory, anti-inflammatory, Th1, Th2, Th17, Th22, and Treg responses, as well as antibody-mediated responses (Gil and Gozalbo 2006; Takeda et al., 2003). After coupling PRRs with their receptors in the fungal cell wall, a wide variety of signal transduction pathways are activated in host cells. This leads to the modulation of the transcription of a large number of immunomodulatory genes, which ultimately dictates the type of immune response that will be mounted against the fungus. Figure 3.1 illustrates the interactions between the immune system of the host and the microflora and *C. albicans* in the gastrointestinal (GI) tract.

It is not clear how the host response contributes to exacerbation of the fungal infection. However, it is known that it depends on a number of interrelated factors. For example, there are inconsistencies regarding the role of the fungus

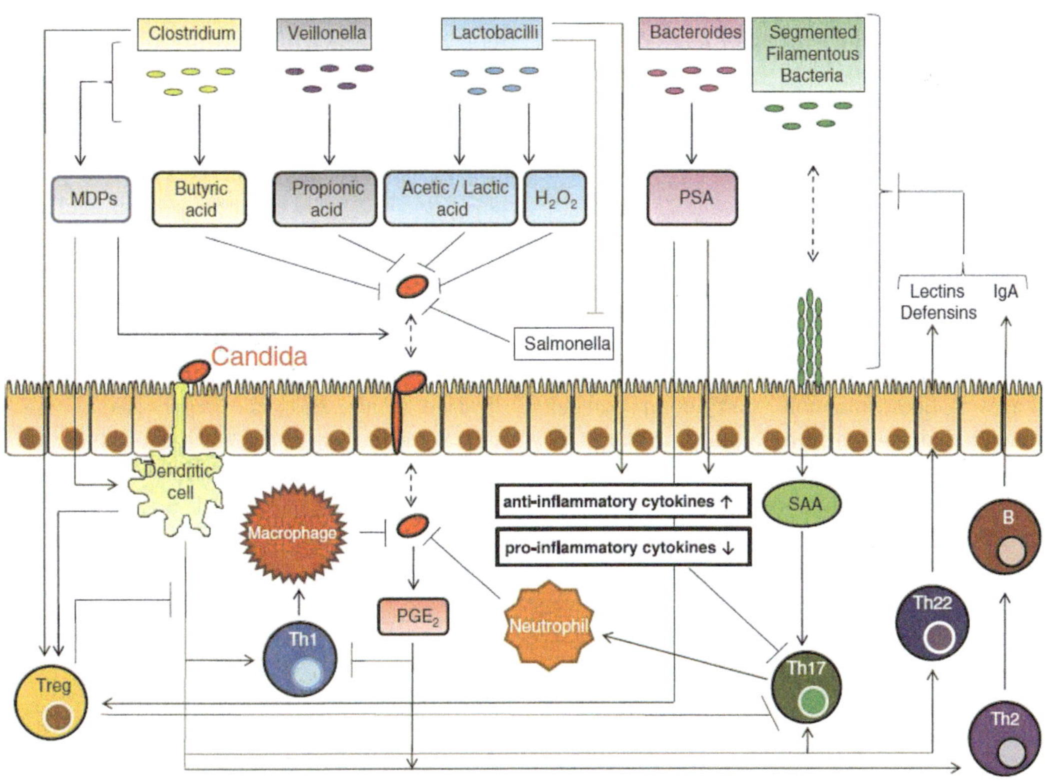

Fig. 3.1 Schematic representation of the important interactions between the immune system of the host, and bacterial microbiota and *C. albicans* in the GI tract. The GI microbiota produce several short-chain fatty acids known as inhibitors of the growth of C. *albicans*, but secrete parallel muramyl dipeptides (MDPs) that improve various virulence factors, including morphological transformation of yeasts to hyphae. The activation of Th17 cells results in the recruitment of neutrophils and macrophages, which share the ability to neutralize *C. albicans*. Macrophages, through the production of prostaglandin E2, prevent the differentiation of Th1 cells in favor of Th2 cells. Dendritic cells play a key role in the differentiation of various types of cells (Treg, Th1, Th2, Th17, and Th22). B lymphocytes, activated by IgA-producing Th2 cells, and epithelial cells, in response to Th22, release defensin. *Fonte: Fabien Cottier • Norman Pavelka* (Cottier and Pavelka 2012)

interactions in inflammation in the host. On one hand, animals that do not have receptors for IL-1, IL-18, or NLRP3 exhibit increased susceptibility to fungal infection in the GI tract. On the other hand, exaggerated inflammatory responses are not associated with increased protection, but rather increased susceptibility to fungal infection, as is seen in patients suffering from immune reconstitution inflammatory syndrome (IRIS) (Singh and Perfect 2007). These apparently contradictory observations point to the fact that the host response to fungal infections does not follow a linear and predictable path, but it is suggested that there is a more complex balance in place to ensure control of the fungal burden and restrict damage to the host tissue (Romani 1999, 2011).

There are barriers, which are comprised of epithelial skin cells that are very close to each other, that block the passage of microorganisms. The cells of the GI tract produce mucus that physically prevents fungal invasion, and removal is possible by the action of intestinal peristalsis (Romani 1999, Romani 2004).

Oral Candidiasis

Oral candidiasis is a common opportunistic infection of the oral cavity and presents similar challenges in both immunologically competent and immunodeficient patients (Samaranayake et al., 2009). Studies have reported that 90 % of patients with acquired immunodeficiency (i.e., HIV) infection develop oropharyngeal, which is characterized by lesions that are pseudomembranous, erythematous or angular cheilitis, during the course of the disease (Repentigny et al., 2004). About 80 % of all fungal infections are caused by *Candida*, typically *C. albicans*. However, *non-albicans Candida*, such as *C. glabrata*, *C. tropicalis*, *C. parapsilosis*, *C. Guilliermondii*, and *C. krusei*, are also pathogenic to humans and have emerged as important opportunistic pathogens of the oral mucosa (Li et al., 2007).

Studies have focused on the interaction of *C. albicans* with macrophages and systemic infections (Herre et al., 2004; Mencacci et al., 2000). Although little is known about the performance of the oral mucosa in the regulation of fungal infections, some studies have contributed to the understanding of pathogen recognition and cell signaling mechanisms in oral epithelium. *C. albicans* interacts with epithelial cells through adhesion, invasion, and induction of cellular damage (Fig. 3.2).

Several advances have been reported in the literature that help to better explain the role of receptor signaling and regulation of immune response against pathogenic fungi in the oral cavity (Graham and Brown 2009; Mencacci et al., 1996). Innate immunity also plays an important role in stimulating the acquired immune response and improves its action against various microorganisms. Innate immunity, which is the first line of defense against microorganisms, includes leukocytes and epithelial barriers.

The interaction between fungi and the host is initiated by cell–cell interactions at the plasma membrane. Several different molecules are found in the walls of fungal cells and serve as molecular patterns (i.e., PAMPs) that are associated with specific pathogens. The PAMPs are recognized by PRRs. The cell wall of most fungi, including *C. albicans*, is composed of a layer of β-(1,3)-glucans linked to β-(1,6)-glucans and chitin, in which the cell wall proteins, and O-linked and N-linked mannans are incorporated. In addition, there are receptors that recognize molecules synthesized by the host, the expression of which indicates cellular damage, known as DAMP (Damage Associated Molecular Patterns).

Mammals have developed a series of PRRs capable of recognizing different molecular fragments that compose the fungal cell wall. PAMPs (Pathogen-associated molecular patterns) for fungi and PRR (Pattern Recognition Receptor) include Toll-like receptors (TLR), C-type lectin receptors (CLRs), Nod-like receptors (NLR) (nucleotide-binding oligomerization domain), and galectin family proteins (Graham and Brown 2009; La Sala et al., 1996). TLRs are a family of evolutionarily conserved signaling receptors that respond to bacterial antigens, fungal and viral. They are found on the cell surface and intracellular membranes and, thus, are capable of recognizing microorganisms different cellular locations intracellular. TLRs induce, among other cellular

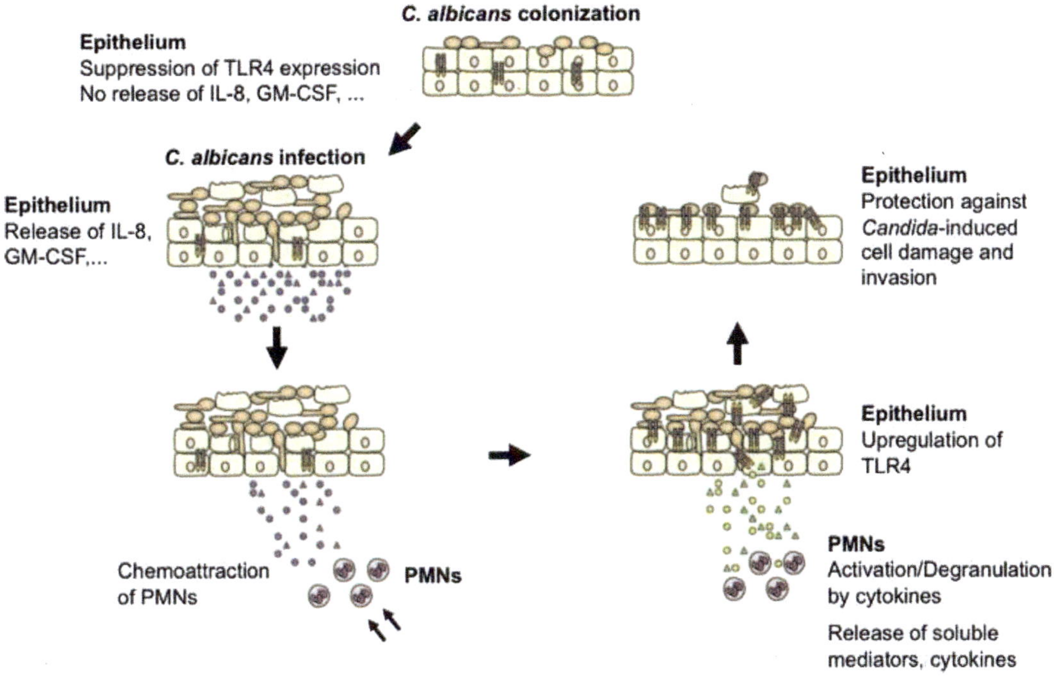

Fig. 3.2 Model of TLR4-mediated and PMN-dependent antifungal defense by the oral epithelium. In general, experimental oral infections can be divided into three phases: an attachment phase, an invasion phase, and a tissue destruction phase. Although *C. albicans* normally exists as a yeast cell, adherent yeast cells rapidly form germ tubes after contact with epithelial cells, and hyphae penetrate the epithelium. Tissue damage is increased dramatically over time, as hyphae penetrate not only the top layer of tissue, but also deeper epithelial cell layers. In contrast, epithelial cells control fungal cell growth and invasion. During colonization of the oral epithelium, *C. albicans* suppresses TLR4 expression and does not induce cytokine production. Infection, particularly in predisposed patients, leads to increased cytokine secretion that recruits and stimulates PMNs at the site of infection. After recruitment, several cytokines, especially TNF, are directly involved in initiating the subsequent PMN-mediated upregulation of epithelial TLR4 through a process that does not require PMN infiltration of the mucosal tissues. Finally, epithelial TLR4 directly protects the oral mucosa from fungal invasion and cell injury, possibly by production of antimicrobial peptides. *Fonte: G. Weindl, J. Wagener, and M. Schaller* (Weindl et al., 2010)

responses, innate immunity, the production of cytokines, chemokines, and endothelial adhesion molecules. They have the ability to recognize a variety of microbial antigens and endogenous factors, presented well, the primary function of acting as receptors sentry to alert the innate immune system signs of infection or tissue damage (Netea et al., 2008).

TLR are expressed on macrophages, dendritic cells, neutrophils, endothelial, and epithelial cells of mucous membranes (Takeda et al., 2003). TLR2, TLR4, TLR6, and TLR9 have been implicated in interactions with fungal sens[aory PAMPs, such as mannans O-linked β-glucans and fungal nucleic acids (Miyazato et al., 2009; Romani et al., 1997).

The main PRRs and their ligands derived from *C. albicans* are shown in Fig. 3.3. Although the main focus of antifungal innate immunity research has been on systemic *Candida* infections, little is known about the role of TLRs in fungal infections located. From studies of fungal infections in knock-out mice deficient in either TLRs or TLR-associated adapter molecules, it appears that specific TLRs, such as TLR2, TLR4, TLR6, and TLR9, play different roles in the activation of the innate immune response. Different research groups have demonstrated divergent roles for TLR2 and TLR4, and their importance in the control of *C. albicans* infection is still uncertain.

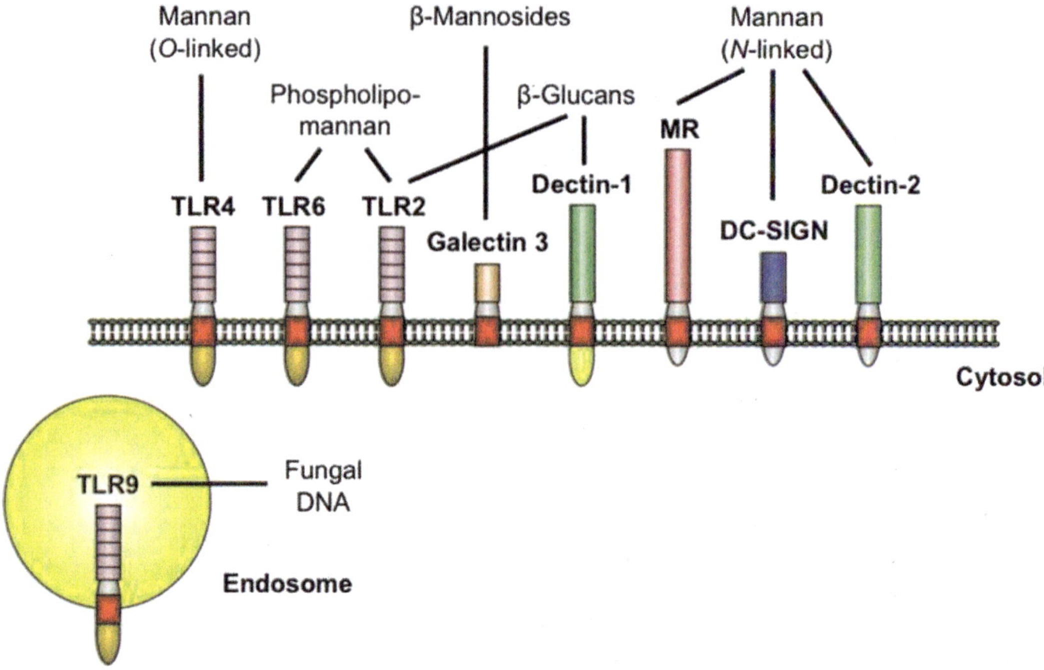

Fig. 3.3 The major PRRs involved in the recognition of specific *C. albicans* PAMPs. Stimulation of the host response by *C. albicans* at the cell membrane is mediated by a limited number of PRRs from the TLR and CLR families. Upon activation, the receptors trigger common adaptor molecules, intracellular pathways, and transcription factors (not shown). However, the specificity of the host response is maintained by the different repertoire of receptors stimulated by certain fungal PAMPs, as well as by the complex interactions between the pathways. The depicted PRRs are predominantly expressed on cells of the myeloid lineage. Oral epithelial cells have been shown to express functional TLR2, TLR4, TLR6, and TLR9, emphasizing the importance of TLRs in the interaction of *C. albicans* and the oral epithelium

NLRs, including Nod1, Nod2, and Nod3 are found intracellularly and recognize peptidoglycan derivatives, microbial cell wall components, and other intracellular signals leading to danger. They activate the host defense through activation of the NF-kB response and inflammatory caspases (Bryant and Fitzgerald 2009). Various NLR family members, including NLRP3 (also known as cryopyrin and NALP3), form a large multiprotein complex called the inflammasome, which activates caspase-1 processing and secretion of IL-1β and IL-18.

C-type lectins (CLRs) are a family of ligand molecules calcium-dependent carbohydrate expressed in the plasma membranes of leukocytes, macrophages, and cells that recognize carbohydrate dendritics, such as mannose, found in the cell walls of microorganisms (Willment and Brown 2008). Several extracellular and transmembrane CLRS, including mannose receptor (MR), Dectin-1, Dectin-2, dendritic cell-specific intercellular adhesion molecule 3-grabbing nonintegrin (DC-SIGN), and macrophage-inducible C-type lectin (Mincle), are involved in antifungal immunity, although their roles are not fully understood. These receptors contribute to the initiation and/or modulation of immune response to this organism.

The MR (CD206) is a prototype type I transmembrane protein and is expressed primarily by macrophages and DCs, and recognize various organisms, including *C. albicans*. After recognition, the carbohydrate receptor mediates internalization of pathogens by phagocytosis, intracellular killing bearing. MR mediates a variety of cellular responses, including activation of NF-kB and production of the cytokines IL-12, IL-8, IL-1ß, IL-6, IL-17, and granulocyte–macrophage colony-stimulating factor (GM-CSF). Moreover, the MR can act as an immunosuppressant based on its ability to inhibit the production of inflammatory cytokines when certain pathogenic fungi are recognized.

Dectin-1 is a type II transmembrane receptor, which belongs to the NK (Natural Killer) cell receptor-like and CLRs. It also synergizes with TLR2- and TLR4-induced signals, inducing tumor necrosis factor (TNF), IL-10, transforming growth factor-β, and maturation of DCs (Herre et al., 2004).

Dectin-2 is a type II transmembrane receptor with a single carbohydrate recognition domain (CRD) and stalk region, but no intracellular signaling motif. Dectin-2 is expressed on macrophages and DCs and is upregulated when these cells are stimulated with particles containing high-mannose structures, such as *C. albicans* hyphae (McGreal et al., 2006).

Oral Mucosal T-Cell Responses to *C. albicans*

Resistance to the fungal infections caused by *C. albicans* requires coordinated action of the innate and adaptive immune responses, during which the activation of systems induces the secretion of a variety of proinflammatory cytokines and expression of costimulatory molecules. Furthermore, the mucosal epithelial cells produce a variety of substances in response to *C. albicans*. Since this kind of microorganism is closely associated with mucosal epithelial cells as a commensal organism, it is important to know the types of substances that are produced.

A better understanding of cytokines is necessary to understand their function and uses in therapy and prophylaxis of fungal infections, if only for their functions and interactions with antifungal drugs. The cytokines produced are derived from the T cells. Two different groups of $CD4^+$ T precursor cells are produced, known as the Th1 and Th2. The differentiation of $CD4^+$ T cells is dependent on the species of *Candida* and the presence of cytokines produced by the local and host immunity. The induction response Th1 cell mediate protection dependent on phagocytes, whose cytokines produced. More important for defense against *C. albicans* are IL-2, IFN-γ, IL-12, and TNF-α. In contrast, Th2 cells produce the cytokine inhibitors, such as IL-4 and IL-10, that are associated with phagocytes and disabling disease progression.

It can be argued that this genetically determined resistance to primary and secondary infections is correlated with the balance occurring between protective Th1 and nonprotective Th2 CD4 cells. However, activation of the innate immune system is not sufficient to control the infection alone, but the important interaction with the adaptive system is needed for the control of infections by *C. albicans*. The acquired immunity correlates with the expression of Th1 at the site or peripheral of the infection. The Th2 response is dependent on the patient's health.

Upon activation of leukocyte populations by *C. albicans*, the first step in activation of the immune response is the release of proinflammatory cytokines, such as TNF-α, IL-1β, IL-6, and IFN-γ (Netea et al., 2008). Proinflammatory cytokines activate macrophages and neutrophils to phagocytose the fungus and release toxic oxygen radicals and nitrogen, thus eliminating the invading pathogen. While macrophages, neutrophils, endothelial cells, fibroblasts, and T and B lymphocytes all secrete TNF-α, however, macrophages are the main sources in vivo. This cytokine exerts multiple biological effects, including cell proliferation and differentiation, apoptosis, cytotoxicity, inflammation, and immunomodulation. In addition, TNF-α also induces the production of other cytokines, such as IL-6 and IL-1, which may participate in the host response during the course of systemic infection by *C. albicans* (Takeda et al., 2003; Underhill et al., 2005). The release of TNF-α by macrophages during the early phase of the inflammatory response to fungus attracts and activates neutrophils to become antifungal effectors.

Even among the Th1 cytokines, IFN-γ is a potent activator of phagocytes. It also acts on cell differentiation. IL-12 is required for optimal Th1 development. The production of IL-4 is dependent on the amount of fungus present in the infection site. IL-10 was first described as a cytokine that had potent anti-inflammatory activity. Th cells are the main inhibitor of the innate immune response, an inflammatory and immunoregulatory.

References

Bryant C, Fitzgerald KA (2009) Molecular mechanisms involved in inflammasome activation. Trends Cell Biol 19(9):455–464

Chapman SW, Sullivan DC, Cleary JD (2008) In search of the holy grail of antifungal therapy. Trans Am Clin Climatol Assoc 119:197–216

Cottier F, Pavelka N (2012) Complexity and dynamics of host–fungal interactions. Immunol Res 53:127–135

Dillon S, Agrawal S, Banerjee K, Letterio J, Denning TL, Oswald-Richter K, Kasprowicz DJ, Kellar K, Pare J, Van Dyke T, Ziegler S, Unutmaz D, Pelendran B (2006) Yeast zymosan, a stimulus for TLR2 and dectin-1, induces regulatory antigen-presenting cells and immunological tolerance. J Clin Invest 116:916–928

Eggimann P, Bille J, Marchetti O (2011) Diagnosis of invasive candidiasis in the ICU. Ann Intensive Care 1:37

Fidel PL Jr, Ginsburg KA, Cutright JL, Wolf NA, Leaman D, Dunlap K, Sobel JD (1997) Vaginal-associated immunity in women with recurrent vulvovaginal candidiasis: evidence for vaginal Th1-type responses following intravaginal challenge with *Candida* antigen. J Infect Dis 176:728–739

Gil ML, Gozalbo D (2006) TLR2, but not TLR4, triggers cytokine production by murine cells in response to *Candida albicans* yeasts and hyphae. Microbes Infect 8(8):2299–2304

Graham LM, Brown GD (2009) The Dectin-2 family of C-type lectins in immunity and homeostasis. Cytokine 48:148–155

Herre J, Marshall AS, Caron E, Edwards AD, Williams DL, Schweighoffer E, Tybulewicz V, Reis e Sousa C, Gordon S, Brown GD (2004) Dectin-1 uses novel mechanisms for yeast phagocytosis in macrophages. Blood 104:4038–4045

La Sala A, Urbani F, Torosantucci A, Cassone A, Ausiello C (1996) Mannoproteins from *Candida albicans* elicit a Th-type-1 cytokine profile in human Candida specific long-term T cell cultures. J Biol Regulat Homeostat Agents 10:8–12

Li L, Redding S, Dongari-Bagtzoglou A (2007) *Candida glabrata*: an emerging oral opportunistic pathogen [review]. J Dent Res 86:204–215

Maródi L, Korchak HM, Johnson Júnior RB (1991) Mechanisms of host defense against Candida species. I. Phagocitosis by monocytes and monocyte-derived macrophages. J Immunol 146(8):2783–2789

McGreal EP, Rosas M, Brown GD, Zamze S, Wong SY, Gordon S, Martinez-Pomares L, Taylor PR (2006) The carbohydrate-recognition domain of Dectin-2 is a C-type lectin with specificity for high mannose. Glycobiology 16:422–430

Mencacci A, Spaccapelo R, Del Sero G, Enssle KH, Cassone A, Bistoni F, Romani L (1996) CD4+ T-helper-cell responses in mice with low-level Candida albicans infection. Infect Immun 64:4907–4914

Mencacci A, Cenci E, Bacci A, Montagnoli C, Bistoni F, Romani L (2000) Cytokines in candidiasis and aspergillosis. Curr Pharm Biotechnol 1(3):235–251

Miceli MH, Díaz JA, Lee SA (2011) Emerging opportunistic yeast infections. Lancet Infect Dis 11:142–151

Miyazato A, Nakamura K, Yamamoto N, Mora-Montes HM, Tanaka M, Abe Y, Tanno D, Inden K, Gang X, Ishii K, Takeda K, Akira S (2009) Toll-like receptor 9-dependent activation of myeloid dendritic cells by deoxynucleic acids from *Candida albicans*. Infect Immun 77(7):3056–3064

Netea MG, Brown GD, Kullberg BJ, Gow NA (2008) An integrated model of the recognition of *Candida albicans* by the innate immune system. Nat Rev Microbiol 6(1):67–78

Odds FC (2003) Antifungal agents: their diversity and increasing sophistication. Mycologist 17:51–55

Repentigny L, Lewandowski D, Jolicoeur P (2004) Immunopathogenesis of oropharyngeal candidiasis in human immunodeficiency virus infection. Clin Microbiol Rev 17(4):729–759

Romani L (1999) Immunity to *Candida albicans*: Th1, Th2 cells and beyond. Curr Opin Microbiol 2:363–367

Romani L (2004) Immunity to fungal infections. Nat Rev Microbiol 4(1):1–13

Romani L (2011) Immunity to fungal infections. Nat Rev Immunol 11(4):275–288

Romani L, Bistoni F, Puccetti P (1997) Initiation of T helper cell immunity to *Candida albicans* by IL-12: the role of neutrophils. Chem Immunol 68:110–135

Samaranayake LP, Keung Leung W, Jin L (2009) Oral mucosal fungal infections. Periodontology 2000 49:39–59

Singh N, Perfect JR (2007) Immune reconstitution syndrome and exacerbation of infections after pregnancy. Clin Infect Dis 45(9):1192–1199

Takeda K, Kaisho T, Akira S (2003) Toll-like receptors. Ann Rev Immunol 21:335–376

Underhill DM, Rossnagle E, Lowell CA, Simmons RM (2005) Dectin-1 activates Syk tyrosine kinase in a dynamic subset of macrophages for reactive oxygen production. Blood 106:2543–2550

Weindl G, Wagener J, Schaller M (2010) Epithelial cells and innate antifungal defense. J Dent Res 89(7):666–675

Willment JA, Brown GD (2008) C-type lectin receptors in antifungal immunity. Trends Microbiol 16:27–32

4 Antifungals for Candidosis Treatment

Ana Maria Trindade Grégio, Flávia Fusco Veiga, Mariana Rinaldi, and Patrícia Vida Cassi Bettega

Abstract

The available treatments for oral candidosis have proved to be more efficacious with the use of new and known antifungal drugs. The success of these is directly related to the correct diagnosis, identification, and correction of etiological factors and the commitment of the patient. In the absence of some of these factors, the antifungal therapy results only in a brief relief from disease, triggering relapses. This chapter presents the main drugs used in the treatment of oral and oropharyngeal candidosis, their functioning in the human body, and their mechanism of action in the destruction of the pathogenic agent.

The available treatments for oral candidosis have been proved to be more efficacious with the use of new and known antifungal drugs.

The success of these is directly related to the correct diagnosis, identification, and correction of etiological factors and the commitment of the patient. In the absence of some of these factors, the antifungal therapy results only in a brief relief from disease, triggering relapses (Akpan and Morgan 2002).

During treatment, harmful habits such as smoking should be completely eliminated or reduced. Oral hygiene needs to be improved, especially in cases of patients that use oral removable prosthesis since disruption of the biofilm produced by *Candida* sp. consists of an important adjunct factor in the healing process (Giannini and Shetty 2011).

For healthy individuals, the treatment of oral candidosis is relatively simple and effective, and the use of topic medications quite suitable. The first chosen drugs are Nystatin oral suspension, clotrimazole tablets, and amphotericin B of oral suspension. For the success of this treatment, proper contact of the oral mucosa with the drug is required (2 min). If the patient is using intraoral devices such as dentures, they must be removed during the application of the drug. The treatment has a variable duration of 7–14 days, continuing for 2–3 days after the disappearance of clinical signs and symptoms of the infection (Li et al. 2014; Melkoumov et al. 2013).

A.M.T. Grégio, BPharm, MSc, PhD (✉)
F.F. Veiga, DDS, MSc • M. Rinaldi, DDS, MSc
P.V.C. Bettega, DDS, MSc
School of Health and Biosciences, Pontifícia Universidade Católica do Paraná, Curitiba, Brazil
e-mail: ana.gregio@pucpr.br

E.A.R. Rosa (ed.), *Oral Candidosis: Physiopathology, Decision Making, and Therapeutics*,
DOI 10.1007/978-3-662-47194-4_4

Topical agents at therapeutic doses have few side effects due to lack of gastrointestinal absorption; however, they contain sucrose, which is cardiogenic, and if used for longer periods, the patient may require adjunct therapy fluorine, as a prevention to the development of caries.

Systemic antifungal such as ketoconazole, fluconazole, and itraconazole have the advantage of once daily dosing and simultaneously treat other fungal infections at multiple body sites. However, these drugs have more side effects, and their selection should consider important interactions with other medicines (Muzyka and Glick 1995).

In immunocompromised patients, such as HIV infected, oral candiosis may lead to secondary complications such as oropharyngeal candidosis. For those at high risk of developing the disease, antifungal prophylaxis is indicated (Vazquez 2010).

Due to the effectiveness of this therapy for the treatment of oropharyngeal candidosis, low mortality, the possibility of interactions with other drugs, and the yearly cost per patient of prophylaxis, the US Public Health Service and the Infectious Disease Society of America do not recommend routine prophylaxis as primary in the United States. There is also a growing concern about azole-resistant fungal strains, as a consequence of chronic suppressive therapy in HIV patients (Pappas et al. 2009; Patel et al. 2012).

This chapter presents the main drugs used in the treatment of oral and oropharyngeal candidosis, their functioning in the human body, and their mechanism of action in the destruction of the pathogenic agent.

Polyenic Agents

This group of drugs is of great clinical use because it presents broad spectrum of activity against common superficial and deep fungal diseases. This class of drugs acts specifically in ergosterol (sterol of fungal cell membrane, absent in animal cells). The drug–ergosterol interaction is able to increase the permeability of the fungal membrane, causing the formation of pores or channels, leading to disturbances in the ionic balance and loss of potassium, sodium, and intracellular ions (Kerridge 1986; Park and Kang 2011).

Amphotericin B

Derived from *Streptomyces nodosus* cultures, microorganisms found in soil (Giannini and Shetty 2011; Vazquez 2010; Pappas et al. 2009; Klotz 2006; Sharon and Fazel 2010; Thompson et al. 2010; Neville et al. 2002). Gold and colleagues discovered this macrolide in 1956. It acts by increasing the permeability of the cell membrane of fungi, leading to loss of cytoplasmic constituents. Depending on the type of fungus, the drug concentration, and the pH of the medium, it presents fungicides and fungistatic functions.

Absorption, Distribution, and Excretion: This drug has little absorption in the skin or mucous membrane, and is held by the gastrointestinal tract. Only a small amount of amphotericin B is available in the bloodstream and has pharmacological action, since over 90 % of it is present in plasma and bind to plasma proteins.

The exact pathway of the drug is unknown; however, it is known that most of it is biotransformed and slowly eliminated through the kidneys. Its features are found in the urine up to 2 months or more after the administration. It displays a plasma half-life of approximately 15 days.

In patients with renal disease, it is not necessary to adjust the dose of this medicine. Approximately 2–5 % of each dose is present in the urine, while individuals are subjected to daily therapy.

Therapeutic Use

Oral solution (trade name suggested Fungizone®). Mouthwash with 1 mL of the solution (100 mg) for 14 days, four times a day, preferably after meals and before bedtime.

In systemic infection, amphotericin B is administered intravenously at doses from 0.4 to 0.6 mg/kg/day for 4 weeks or more (trade name suggested Anforicin B® 50 mg).

Adverse Effects:
Nausea, vomiting, rash, diarrhea, and gastrointestinal disorders. Intravenously, amphotericin B is the most toxic antibiotic in use currently and may lead to hypotension, fever, nausea, abdominal pain, and more. In this via, all patients show some degree of nephrotoxicity and may have thereby stopped treatment. For individuals with preexisting liver problems, undergoing treatment for over a month, the monitoring of liver function is indicated.

Amphotericin B has no significant drug interactions.

Nystatin

Discovered in the 1950s, by the New York State Health Laboratory, it was the first effective treatment for the cure of oral candidosis (Giannini and Shetty 2011; Melkoumov et al. 2013; Muzyka and Glick 1995; Vazquez 2010; Pappas et al. 2009; Park and Kang 2011; Klotz 2006; Neville et al. 2002; Greenspan 1994). Derived from *Streptomyces noursei* culture, this macrolide resembles in its structure the amphotericin B. It can be both fungistatic and fungicidal and has reduced activity compared to amphotericin B. It is the most used for oral candidosis and used in immunocompromised patients as prophylactic treatment.

Because of its bitter taste, this drug is difficult to be accepted by patients. Laboratories add certain amount of sucrose and flavoring to its formulation. Therefore, patients with xerostomia, and because of this, oral candidosis, are more susceptible to the development of caries.

Absorption, Distribution, and Excretion:
Poorly absorbed by the gastrointestinal tract, skin, and mucous membranes, the action of this drug starts as soon as it comes in contact with the pathogen, in oral or intestinal cavity.

Significant concentrations of nystatin may occasionally appear in the plasma of patients with renal impairment during oral therapy with standard doses.

After oral administration, most nystatin is eliminated unchanged in the feces. Due to its high systemic toxicity, nystatin is not administered parenterally.

Therapeutic Use:
Oral solution (trade name suggested Micostatin®). In adults and children mouthwash with subsequent swallowing of 4 to 6 mL of the solution (1: 100,000 IU).

Neonates and preterm with low birth weight should receive 1 mL of this solution. Lactating children should receive 2 mL, which can be applied to the flexible stem of aid or gauze. This treatment must be continued for 14 days, four times a day, preferably after meals and before bedtime.

Tablets (brand name suggested Mycostatin Tablet®). One or two tablets (200,000–400,000 IU) dissolved in the mouth four times daily for 14 days.

Adverse Effects:
Nausea, diarrhea, and vomiting at high doses of the drug.

Nystatin liposomal (encapsulated in liposomes) has low systemic cytotoxicity, showing more effectiveness in cases of resistance to amphotericin B.

The polyene derivative, despite its high antifungal activity, has a poor intestinal absorption, which makes its use in the treatment of oral candidosis limited.

Cases of resistance to the use of polyenic are rare; however, if it occurs, it is due to a reduction of the amount of ergosterol constituent of the fungal cell wall.

It has no drug interaction with other drugs.

Imidazole and Triazole Agents

Developed in 1970, these drugs inhibit sterol 14-α-demethylase, a small set of enzymes dependant on cytochrome P450. There is blockade of ergosterol production, causing accumulation of substances and impairment of the functions responsible for fungal growth (Cupp-Vickery et al. 2001).

These agents are also capable of inhibiting the transformation of yeast cells of *Candida* spp. in hyphae, which makes the microorganism less aggressive (Park and Kang 2011).

Ketoconazole

It was the first drug used for the treatment of systemic candidosis orally (Giannini and Shetty 2011; Muzyka and Glick 1995; Vazquez 2010; Pappas et al. 2009; Park and Kang 2011; Klotz 2006; Sharon and Fazel 2010; Thompson et al. 2010; Neville et al. 2002; Greenspan 1994; Van Roey et al. 2004). Only in rare cases of resistance to other antifungals the prescription of ketoconazole is necessary.

According to the Food and Drug Administration (FDA), ketoconazole cannot be used as initial therapy for the treatment of oral candidosis. If it is used for more than 2 weeks by the patient, liver function studies are recommended, since 1 in 10,000 develops idiosyncratic drug toxicity.

Responsible for inhibiting the production of estradiol and testosterone, it may cause abnormalities in the menstrual cycle and gynecomastia.

Absorption, Distribution, and Excretion: Well absorbed by the gastrointestinal tract, since its content remains acid. Drugs that increase gastric pH (antacids and antihistamines), rifampicin and antagonists of the histamine H2 receptor and omeprazole lower its absorption.

Distributed to the tissue and tissue fluids, it has poor penetration into the central nervous system, except when used at high doses. It is extensively metabolized by the liver and excreted in bile and urine, where the active drug concentrations are very low. In the blood, 84 % of ketoconazole bind to plasmatic proteins (albumin); 15 % to erythrocytes and remains in the free form.

The metabolism of this drug is not altered by azotemia (biochemical alteration in the compounds of nitrogen/nitrogen in renal function), by hemodialysis, or peritoneal dialysis. The presence of moderate hepatic impairment has no effect on its blood concentration.

Ketoconazole inhibits the metabolism of cyclosporine, phenytoin, sulfonylureas, warfarin and antihistamines, terfenadine, and astemizole. Isoniazid, antibiotic used to treat tuberculosis, increases its metabolism.

The bioavailability of the drug is reduced in patients with achlorhydria, especially those with AIDS, who must ingest acidifying agents like orange juice prior to the administration of ketoconazole.

Interactions of ketoconazole with macrolide antibiotics, enhancing agents of gastrointestinal motility and some antihistamines, may lead to cardiac arrhythmias with potentially life threatening.

Clotrimazole

More tolerated by patients because it has better taste than the nystatin (Giannini and Shetty 2011; Muzyka and Glick 1995; Pappas et al. 2009; Park and Kang 2011; Sharon and Fazel 2010; Thompson et al. 2010; Neville et al. 2002; Greenspan 1994; Sangeorzan et al. 1994).

Absorption, Distribution, and Excretion: Its absorption by the gastrointestinal tract is poor, being insoluble in aqueous medium. It is metabolized by the liver and excreted with the feces together with the unabsorbed drug.

Therapeutic Use: Tablets (brand name suggested Mycelex oral tablets®). One tablet (10 mg) dissolved slowly in the mouth, five times a day, for 14 days.

Adverse Effects: Nausea and vomiting. Patients with hepatic impairment should be evaluated periodically, because in 15 % of patients treated with this drug there was a slight increase in the number of liver enzymes. No significant drug interactions.

Itraconazole

It is one of the newest synthetic triazole agents, being less toxic than other antifungal (Giannini and Shetty 2011; Muzyka and Glick 1995; Vazquez 2010; Pappas et al. 2009; Park and Kang 2011; Sharon and Fazel 2010; Thompson et al. 2010; Neville et al. 2002; Greenspan 1994).

Absorption, Distribution, and Excretion:
This drug has good absorption by the gastrointestinal tract when taken with meals. Metabolized primarily in the liver and partly eliminated in bile.

Exhibits high plasma protein binding (99 %) and has a prolonged half-life, 20 h after a single dose and up to 60 h at steady state. When administered orally, its half-life is 36 h.

Similarly to ketoconazole, itraconazole also requires low gastric pH for bioavailability.

Therapeutic Use:
Oral suspension (trade name suggested Sporanox® oral suspension). Mouthwashes followed by swallowing with 10 mL of the solution (100 mg) for 1 or 2 weeks.

Adverse Effects:
Nausea, diarrhea, and vomiting. Hypocalcemia, hypertension, rash, and heart failure in susceptible patients. There are rare cases of hepatotoxicity.

Few drug interactions have been reported in the literature using the itraconazole. Some can be considered serious and / or life threatening, when the drug is administered in doses of 200 mg together with terfenadine, astemizole, oral triazolam, oral midazolam, and cisapride.

Fluconazole

Very effective medication due to the greater specificity than ketoconazole in the treatment of oral candidosis, especially in immunocompromised and immunosuppressed individuals (Giannini and Shetty 2011; Muzyka and Glick 1995; Vazquez 2010; Pappas et al. 2009; Park and Kang 2011; Klotz 2006; Sharon and Fazel 2010; Thompson et al. 2010; Neville et al. 2002; Sangeorzan et al. 1994; Bozzette 2005; Hamza et al. 2008; Millon et al. 1994; Nairy et al. 2011; Neoh et al. 2011; Reboli et al. 2007; Rex et al. 1995; Vazquez et al. 2006). In HIV seropositive patients, it is also used as prophylaxis against candidosis weekly.

Absorption, Distribution, and Excretion:
Is well absorbed by the gastrointestinal tract by binding poorly to plasmatic proteins. It has rapid diffusion in body fluids such as saliva and sputum. After 2 h of oral administration, its maximum plasma concentration occurs. It has long plasma half-life of 20–50 h in adults and 17 h for children. It has high bioavailability without relying on gastric pH.

It is eliminated virtually unchanged by the kidney (90 %) and the feces (10 %).

Therapeutic Use:
Oral tablets (trade name suggested Diflucan® tablets.) Two tablets (200 mg) on day one, and then one tablet (100 mg) daily, for 7–14 days.

Adverse Effects:
Nausea, vomiting, headache, diarrhea, rash, abdominal pain, and rare cases of hepatotoxicity.

Drug interactions are reported for some hypoglycemic agents, anticoagulants, and anticoa anticonvulsants (phenytoin derivatives).

There is a concern about the use of fluconazole as primary agent due to its potential for the development of strains resistant to azoles.

Posaconazole

Available in Europe since 2005, it was approved by the FDA in 2006 for oropharyngeal candidosis and cases of resistance to itraconazole and/or fluconazole (Giannini and Shetty 2011; Muzyka and Glick 1995; Vazquez 2010; Pappas et al. 2009; Park and Kang 2011; Klotz 2006; Sharon and Fazel 2010; Thompson et al. 2010; Neville et al.

2002; Vazquez et al. 2006; Andes et al. 2004; Ianas et al. 2007; Nagappan and Deresinski 2007). Suitable also as prophylactic therapy of invasive fungal disease in immunosuppressed patients.

For the treatment of oropharyngeal candidosis in HIV, a study demonstrated the pozaconazol to be as effective and safe as fluconazole, when administered at the same dose and duration of treatment. Posaconazole was also shown to be more effective against relapse after completion of treatment (Vazquez 2010).

It has a broad spectrum against filamentous fungi and various types of yeast, having a structure similar to itraconazole. It is available as an oral suspension, making it well-tolerated by patients. As a higher cost drug, it is not used in the routine treatment of oral candidosis, except in cases of resistance to fluconasol.

Absorption, Distribution, and Excretion:
The gastro-intestinal absorption is inadequate and it is optimized when the drug is administered concomitantly with high fat meals or a liquid nutritional supplement. It is affected in the presence of gastrointestinal mucositis and diarrhea.

It has high plasm protein binding (98 %), which gives good tissue distribution. It has plasma half-life of 20–66 h.

Metabolized by the liver and eliminated unchanged in feces (66 %) and urine (14 %).

Therapeutic Use
Oral suspension 40 mg/mL (suggested trade name: Noxafil®). For oropharyngeal candidosis it is administered on the first day of therapy 100 mg two times a day and on the second day from 1 to 100 mg daily for 13 days.

For immunosuppressed, with indication prophylaxis oral candidosis, 200 mg of the drug should be administered three times a day.

Regarding the azole-resistant patients, the dosage is 400 mg two times a day. The duration of therapy depends on the clinical response to treatment.

No dose adjustment is required for geriatric patients and adolescents, and no dose reduction is required for patients with renal or hepatic insufficiency.

No drug clearance during hemodialysis.

The safety and efficacy of posaconazole use are not well established in children under the age of 13 years.

The biggest advantage of this drug compared to amphotericin B is its lower toxicity.

Adverse Effects:
Nausea, vomiting, diarrhea, headache, abdominal pain, dizziness, elevated transaminase and enzymes in the liver, hyperbilirubinemia, and rashes.

Contraindication:
Patients with hypersensitivity to the drug or any of its constituent.

Due to the inhibition of hepatic CYP3A4, posaconazole may cause drug interactions with other drugs metabolized by the same enzyme.

It presents interaction with antivirals, chemotherapeutic agents, and benzodiazepines.

Miconazole

First antifungal imidazole derivative, with topical and parenteral indications (Giannini and Shetty 2011; Muzyka and Glick 1995; Vazquez 2010; Pappas et al. 2009; Park and Kang 2011; Sharon and Fazel 2010; Thompson et al. 2010; Neville et al. 2002; Van Roey et al. 2004; Ahmed et al. 2012; Bensadoun et al. 2008; Collins et al. 2011; Lalla and Bensadoun 2011; Pemberton et al. 2004; Vazquez and Sobel 2012).

There is no systemic indication for this drug anymore due to reports of its interaction with other medicines. It has a half short plasma life and needs to be administered every 8 h. It is not inactivated in the liver and it does not reach the central nervous system.

Outside the United States, miconazole oral gel (brand name Daktarin® oral gel 40 mg) has been used for the treatment of fungal and gastrointestinal infections since early 1977.

Therapeutic Indication:
6–24-month babies: ¼ teaspoon (1.25 mL) gel applied to the affected areas with flexible stem of aid or gauze, four times a day. The gel should not

be swallowed immediately, but kept in the mouth as long as possible.

Adults and 2 years or older children: ½ teaspoon (2.5 mL) gel applied on the affected areas with flexible stem of aid or gauze, four times a day. The gel should not be swallowed immediately, but kept in the mouth as long as possible.

Treatment should be maintained for at least a week after the disappearance of symptoms. Some patients may require a longer period of treatment.

The use of miconazole oral gel for oropharyngeal candidosis presents limitations because the small contact of the drug with the oral mucosa, thus requiring multiple daily applications for a successful treatment.

As a result, a mucoadhesive tablet for miconazole base was recently approved in the United States and in Europe. It promotes release of the drug over a long period of time in the oral cavity with a single daily application.

Absorption, Distribution and Excretion:
Most of the miconazole tablet is metabolized by the liver and excreted in the urine.

Indications:
In the United States, for the treatment of oropharyngeal candidosis for adults and adolescents older than 16 years. In Europe, for the treatment of immunocompromised patients with oral candidosis.

The tablets may also be indicated for cases of dry mouth, oral ulcers, and patients who are resistant to fluconazole, in cases of mild to moderate oropharyngeal candidosis.

Contraindications:
Miconazole patients with hypersensitivity to any drug or component and milk protein; total prosthesis users or upper partials in region of the canine fossa, and under 16 years of age young people, risk of shock.

Disadvantage of use: High cost of the drug.

Therapeutic use: Tablets 50 mg mucoadhesive (Loramyc® in Europe; Oravig® in the United States).

The tablet is applied in the morning after oral hygiene in the region of upper canine fossa with lightweight digital compression, for 30 s.

After humidifying the tablet with saliva, the drug begins to be released slowly in the oral cavity for a period of 6 h. If there is no good grip or it releases in the oral mucosa during this period, a new miconazole tablet should be applied.

Patients can eat normally during the use of miconazole tablet. The product should not be chewed, crushed, or swallowed.

Adverse Effects:
Miconazole tablet should be used with caution in patients with hepatic impairment.

Patients undergoing continuous treatment with anticoagulants such as Warfarin may have bleeding as a result of drug interaction between these drugs. Those using antihistamines, anxiolytics, and cyclosporine should be orientated about the possible deleterious effects of this association.

There is no dose adjustment for patients with renal insufficiency.

Echinocandins

New antifungal class approved by the FDA, formed during the fermentation of fungus *Aspergillus nidulans* var. *echinulatus* (Pappas et al. 2009; Park and Kang 2011).

They have a different action mechanism from other antifungal agents as they inhibit the type 1,3-linked β-D-glucan, responsible for the production of component of the fungus cell wall and for the maintenance of its osmotic balance. The absence of these links in mammalian cells justifies the minimal toxicity of echinocandins.

Caspofungin, micafungin, and anidulafungin are available for use intravenously, indicated for more severe cases of oral candidosis.

There is no indication for use of these drugs in the pediatric clinic.

Caspofungin

Approved by the FDA in 2001. Indicated for patients with severe fungal infection, intolerant to amphotericin glycine B or azoles (Pappas et al. 2009; Park and Kang 2011; Thompson et al. 2010; Hoang 2001; Arathoon et al. 2002).

Therapeutic Use:
Vial of 50 and 75 mg (trade name suggested Cancidas®). Application of 75 mg intravenously on the first day of treatment, followed by doses of 50 mg in the following days.

Adverse Effects:
Exantema, facial sweating, itching, fever, and headache. Phlebitis at the infusion site and a reversible increase in liver enzyme levels may occur. It is not nephrotoxic.

Caspofungin has few significant drug interactions, as it is neither a substrate nor an inhibitor of P-450cytochromes. It may have reduced efficacy when administered concomitantly with carbamazepine, phenytoin, phenobarbital, and dexamethasone. Coadministration with rifampicin may lead to an increase or decrease of the levels of caspofungin.

Degraded mainly in the liver. Small amount is excreted in the bile and urine.

Micafungin

Its use was approved in 2005 by the FDA (Pappas et al. 2009; Park and Kang 2011; Morrison 2006).

Therapeutic Use:
Vial of 50 and 150 mg (trade name suggested Mycamine®). Application of 50–150 mg intravenously daily.

Adverse Effects:
Tremors, backache, and, to a lesser extent, hypocalcemia.

Degraded mainly in the liver and excreted in bile and inactive form urine.

It presents fewer drug interactions than caspofungin.

Anidulafungin

It has a high antifungal potential against some species of candidosis, including those resistant to fluconasol, amphotericin B, or other echinocandins (Pappas et al. 2009; Park and Kang 2011; Thompson et al. 2010; Neoh et al. 2011; Reboli et al. 2007; Ruhnke et al. 2012). It is slowly degraded in the blood, undergoing a biotransformation process rather than being metabolized.

Therapeutic Use:
Vial of 50 mg (trade name suggested Eraxis®). Application of 100 mg intravenously daily.

Adverse Effects:
Hypotension, vomiting, constipation, nausea, fever, hypocalcemia, and elevation of hepatic enzymes.

References

Ahmed TA, El-Say KM et al (2012) Miconazole nitrate oral disintegrating tablets: in vivo performance and stability study. Clin Infect Dis 54(10):1480–1484

Akpan A, Morgan R (2002) Oral candidiasis. Postgrad Med J 78(922):455–459

Andes D, Marchillo K et al (2004) Pharmacodynamics of a new triazole, posaconazole, in a murine model of disseminated candidiasis. Antimicrob Agents Chemother 48(1):137–142

Arathoon EG, Gotuzzo E, Noriega LM, Berman RS, DiNubile MJ, Sable CA (2002) Randomized, double-blind, multicenter study of caspofungin versus amphotericin B for treatment of oropharyngeal and esophageal candidiases. Antimicrob Agents Chemother 46(2):451–457

Bensadoun RJ, Daoud J et al (2008) Comparison of the efficacy and safety of miconazole 50-mg mucoadhesive buccal tablets with miconazole 500-mg gel in the treatment of oropharyngeal candidiasis: a prospective, randomized, single-blind, multicenter, comparative, phase III trial in patients treated with radiotherapy for head and neck cancer. Cancer 112(1):204–211

Bozzette SA (2005) Fluconazole prophylaxis in HIV disease, revisited. Clin Infect Dis 41(10):1481–1482

Collins CD, Cookinham S et al (2011) Management of oropharyngeal candidiasis with localized oral miconazole therapy: efficacy, safety, and patient acceptability. Patient Prefer Adherence 5:369–374

Cupp-Vickery JR, Garcia C, Hofacre A, McGee-Estrada K (2001) Ketoconazole-induced conformational changes in the active site of cytochrome P450eryF. J Mol Biol 311(1):101–110

Giannini PJ, Shetty KV (2011) Diagnosis and management of oral candidiasis. Otolaryngol Clin North Am 44(1):231–240, vii

Greenspan D (1994) Treatment of oropharyngeal candidiasis in HIV-positive patients. J Am Acad Dermatol 31(3 Pt 2):S51–S55

Hamza OJ, Matee MI et al (2008) Single-dose fluconazole versus standard 2-week therapy for oropharyngeal candidiasis in HIV-infected patients: a randomized, double-blind, double-dummy trial. Clin Infect Dis 47(10):1270–1276

Hoang A (2001) Caspofungin acetate: an antifungal agent. Am J Health Syst Pharm 58(13):1206–1214

Ianas V, Matthias KR et al (2007) Role of posaconazole in the treatment of oropharyngeal candidiasis. Ther Clin Risk Manag 3(4):533–542

Kerridge D (1986) Mode of action of clinically important antifungal drugs. Adv Microb Physiol 27:1–72

Klotz SA (2006) Oropharyngeal candidiasis: a new treatment option. Clin Infect Dis 42(8):1187–1188

Lalla RV, Bensadoun RJ (2011) Miconazole mucoadhesive tablet for oropharyngeal candidiasis. Expert Rev Anti Infect Ther 9(1):13–17

Li D et al (2014) Efficacy and safety of probiotics in the treatment of Candida-associated stomatitis. Mycoses 57(3):141–146

Melkoumov A, Goupil M et al (2013) Nystatin nanosizing enhances in vitro and in vivo antifungal activity against Candida albicans. J Antimicrob Chemother 68(9):2099–2105

Millon L, Manteaux A et al (1994) Fluconazole-resistant recurrent oral candidiasis in human immunodeficiency virus-positive patients: persistence of Candida albicans strains with the same genotype. J Clin Microbiol 32(4):1115–1118

Morrison VA (2006) Echinocandin antifungals: review and update. Expert Rev Anti Infect Ther 4(2):325–342

Muzyka BC, Glick M (1995) A review of oral fungal infections and appropriate therapy. J Am Dent Assoc 126(1):63–72

Nagappan V, Deresinski S (2007) Reviews of anti-infective agents: posaconazole: a broad-spectrum triazole antifungal agent. Clin Infect Dis 45(12):1610–1617

Nairy HM, Charyulu NR et al (2011) A pseudo-randomised clinical trial of in situ gels of fluconazole for the treatment of oropharyngeal candidiasis. Trials 12:99

Neoh CF, Liew D et al (2011) Cost-effectiveness analysis of anidulafungin versus fluconazole for the treatment of invasive candidiasis. J Antimicrob Chemother 66(8):1906–1915

Neville BW, Damm DD, Allen CM, Bouquot JE (2002) Fungal and protozoal diseases. In: Neville BW, Damm DD, Allen CM, Bouquot JE (eds) Oral & maxillofacial pathology, 2nd edn. W.B. Saunders Company, Philadelphia, pp 189–211

Pappas PG, Kauffman CA, Andes D, Benjamin DK Jr, Calandra TF, Edwards JE Jr, Filler SG, Fisher JF, Kullberg BJ, Ostrosky-Zeichner L, Reboli AC, Rex JH, Walsh TJ, Sobel JD (2009) Infectious Diseases Society of America. Clinical practice guidelines for the management of candidiasis: 2009 update by the Infectious Diseases Society of America. Clin Infect Dis 48(5):503–535

Park NH, Kang MOK (2011) Antifungal and antiviral agents. In: Mariotti A, Dowd FJ, Johnson B, Yagiela JA (eds) Pharmacology and therapeutics for dentistry, 6th edn. Mosby Inc. an affiliate of Elsevier Inc, Maryland Heights, pp 640–657

Patel PK, Erlandsen JE et al (2012) The changing epidemiology of oropharyngeal candidiasis in patients with HIV/AIDS in the era of antiretroviral therapy. AIDS Res Treat 2012:262471

Pemberton MN, Oliver RJ et al (2004) Miconazole oral gel and drug interactions. Br Dent J 196(9):529–531

Reboli AC, Rotstein C et al (2007) Anidulafungin versus fluconazole for invasive candidiasis. N Engl J Med 356(24):2472–2482

Rex JH, Rinaldi MG et al (1995) Resistance of Candida species to fluconazole. Antimicrob Agents Chemother 39(1):1–8

Ruhnke M, Paiva JA et al (2012) Anidulafungin for the treatment of candidaemia/invasive candidiasis in selected critically ill patients. Clin Microbiol Infect 18(7):680–687

Sangeorzan JA, Bradley SF et al (1994) Epidemiology of oral candidiasis in HIV-infected patients: colonization, infection, treatment, and emergence of fluconazole resistance. Am J Med 97(4):339–346

Sharon V, Fazel N (2010) Oral candidiasis and angular cheilitis. Dermatol Ther 23(3):230–242

Thompson GR 3rd, Patel PK et al (2010) Oropharyngeal candidiasis in the era of antiretroviral therapy. Oral Surg Oral Med Oral Pathol Oral Radiol Endod 109(4):488–495

Van Roey J, Haxaire M et al (2004) Comparative efficacy of topical therapy with a slow-release mucoadhesive buccal tablet containing miconazole nitrate versus systemic therapy with ketoconazole in HIV-positive patients with oropharyngeal candidiasis. J Acquir Immune Defic Syndr 35(2):144–150

Vazquez JA (2010) Optimal management of oropharyngeal and esophageal candidiasis in patients living with HIV infection. HIV AIDS (Auckl) 2:89–101

Vazquez JA, Sobel JD (2012) Miconazole mucoadhesive tablets: a novel delivery system. Clin Infect Dis 54(10):1480–1484

Vazquez JA, Skiest DJ et al (2006) A multicenter randomized trial evaluating posaconazole versus fluconazole for the treatment of oropharyngeal candidiasis in subjects with HIV/AIDS. Clin Infect Dis 42(8): 1179–1186

Acute Oral Erythematous Candidosis

5

Cristiane Yumi Koga Ito, Jorgiana Sangalli, and Daniel Freitas Alves Pereira

Abstract

Acute erythematous candidiasis (EC) is cited as the most frequent clinical manifestation among AIDS patients, after pseudomembranous form. Among HIV-positive patients, it was reported as the most commonly observed oromucosal lesion. Higher prevalence of this condition was observed in patients with CD4/CD8 ratio <0.30 and CD4 levels ≤200 cells/mm. Based on these evidences, the presence of EC has been suggested as a marker to diagnose the immune status of HIV-infected individuals.

Acute erythematous candidiasis (EC) is frequently cited as the most frequent clinical manifestation among AIDS patients, after pseudomembranous form (Tirwomwe et al. 2007). Among HIV-positive patients, it was reported as the most commonly observed oromucosal lesion (Gaurav et al. 2011; Bodhade et al. 2011; Sharma et al. 2006). Higher prevalence of this condition was observed in patients with CD4/CD8 ratio <0.30 (Gaurav et al. 2011) and CD4 levels ≤200 cells/mm (Gonçalves et al. 2013). Based on these evidences, the presence of EC has been suggested as a marker to diagnose the immune status of HIV-infected individuals.

Decrease in the prevalence of erythematous candidiasis has been reported after HAART- era in several places worldwide (Gonçalves et al. 2013; Lourenço et al. 2011; Gaurav et al. 2011). Percentages of erythematous candidiasis occurrence among HIV-positive patients undergoing HAART varies from 7 % to 16 % (Gaitan Cepeda et al. 2008). Some studies observed that HAART promoted an overall reduction in the occurrence of HIV-associated oral lesions and erythematous candidiasis was the clinical form that decreased most (Lourenço et al. 2011).

However, this reduction tendency was not observed in all populations. Previous study reported that the prevalence of EC among pediatric Nigerian patients was not reduced by HAART (Adebola et al. 2012). Also, in a Spanish cohort

C.Y.K. Ito (✉)
Institute of Science and Technology, Oral Biopathology Program and Department of Environmental Engineering, Universidade Estadual Paulista/UNESP, São José dos Campos, Brazil
e-mail: cristiane@ict.unesp.br

J. Sangalli • D.F.A. Pereira
Institute of Science and Technology, Oral Biopathology Graduate Program, Universidade Estadual Paulista/UNESP, São José dos Campos, Brazil

E.A.R. Rosa (ed.), *Oral Candidosis: Physiopathology, Decision Making, and Therapeutics*, DOI 10.1007/978-3-662-47194-4_5 of HIV-positive patients, no reduction of EC was observed after the introduction of HAART (Ceballos-Salobreña et al. 2004).

EC is also frequently observed among end-stage renal disease patients (Thorman et al. 2009; Al-Mohaya et al. 2009) and type 2 diabetes mellitus, representing a challenge for the health maintenance of these patients. Acute erythematous candidiasis associated to hypopharyngeal lesions was reported in patients under treatment with topical intranasal steroids (Kyrmizakis et al. 1999).

Acute erythematous candidiasis clinically presents as localized erythema. It is usually associated to burning sensation and loss of filiform papillae at tongue dorsum (Neville et al. 2009). Although the palate or buccal mucosa may be involved, the most common site of infection is the dorsum of the tongue (Ellepola and Samaranayake 2000; Farah et al. 2010). This variant was also referred as "antibiotic sore mouth," due to its association with chronic use of broad-spectrum antibiotics (Soysa et al. 2008) and corticosteroids (Ellepola and Samaranayake 2001). The use of broad-spectrum antibiotics facilitates the overgrowth of *C. albicans* by suppressing the normal oral bacterial microflora (Williams et al. 2011). The clinical presentation of erythematous tongue with papillary atrophy also occurs in association with other disorders, including iron deficiency anemia, vitamin B12 deficiency, and poorly controlled diabetes *mellitus* and accurate differential diagnosis is necessary (Giannini and Shetty 2011).

The diagnosis of candidiasis is based on clinical findings, and it is confirmed by the identification of blastospores and pseudohyphae in stained smears sampled from the lesion, by the identification of colonies cultured on Sabouraud culture medium or by histological examination (Samaranayake 2006; Worthington et al. 2007; Scully 2004).

The smear is valuable for differentiating between yeast and hyphae forms, but it is less sensitive than culture methods (Williams and Lewis 2000). Due to the lower number of *Candida* cells isolated from erythematous candidiasis lesions when compared to pseudomembranous form, negative results are occasionally obtained when direct examination is used (Terai and Shimahara 2009). In the diagnosis of erythematous candidiasis, examinations are reported to yield false-negative results in 25 % of culture tests and 42.5 % of microscopic examinations (Terai and Shimahara 2009). For this reason, more recently, the combination of fluorescent staining (Fungiflora Y) and observation using a portable fluorescent microscope was suggested for the diagnosis of oral erythematous candidiasis (Okamoto et al. 2013).

Diagnosis of erythematous candidiasis should be clinically differentiated from thermal traumatic lesions, erosive lichen planus and lichenoid reactions, lupus erythematosis, erythema multiforme, pernicious anemia and epithelial dysplasia (Farah et al. 2000).

Due to the opportunistic nature of the disease, the priority in the treatment of oral candidiasis is the resolution of any identifiable predisposing factor. Therefore, acquiring a complete medical history is an essential element for the selection of the treatment (Krishnan 2012).

For patients with prosthesis-associated acute erythematous candidiasis, besides correction of inadequate devices, the improvement of hygiene is an important step of the treatment. The prescription of a denture cleaner with antifungal properties, such as 0.2 % chlorhexidine digluconate, associated to the removal of the dentures at night is the standard protocol (Farah et al. 2010). The xerostomia caused by medication or underlying disease may be controlled by saliva substitutes (Gonsalves et al. 2008).

Some predisposing factors are difficult or impossible to eradicate, such as occurrence of leukemia or AIDS. In such cases, prophylactic reduction in oral levels of *Candida* plays an important role (Lalla et al. 2013). Also in these cases, the reduction may be achieved by hygiene practices, including toothbrushing and the use of antimicrobial mouthwash.

Several mouthwashes have anti-*Candida* activity, including those with triclosan, chlorhexidine digluconate, and formulations containing essential oils (Pusateri et al. 2009). The formulations with natural plant extracts usually contain thymol, eucalyptol, or bioflavonoids (Fine 1988).

The anti-*Candida* activity of these compounds is related to the rupture of cell membrane or enzyme inhibition. Higher efficacy of commercial mouthwashes (Corsodyl, Listerine, and Oraldene) on biofilms in vitro when compared to azole antifungal agents was previously reported (Ramage et al. 2011) and corroborates its prescription in cases of oral candidal infections.

The most commonly used classes of conventional antifungal drugs are the polyenes and azoles. Polyenes class includes amphotericin B and nystatin. They act by direct binding with the ergosterol in fungal cell membrane. The binding polyene-ergosterol induces leakage of cytoplasmic contents leading to fungal cell death (Sanglard and Bille 2002). However, polyenes at therapeutic concentrations exhibit a higher degree of toxicity in humans. Moreover, their use is limited due to the poor intestinal absorption. Topical application in the form of lozenges and oral suspensions are most commonly used for the treatment of oral fungal infection.

Azole antifungals show fungistatic activity rather than fungicidal (Andes 2003). The mechanism of action is most frequently lanosterol demethylase enzyme inhibition, which is a cytochrome P-4503A-dependent enzyme involved in the synthesis of ergosterol (Sanglard and Bille 2002). After depletion of ergosterol from yeast cells, inhibition of fungal growth and impaired membrane permeability are observed (Nimmi et al. 2010).

Itraconazole and fluconazole are most frequently administered for the treatment of oral candidiasis and have the advantage of good intestinal absorption. Furthermore, fluconazole is secreted in saliva at high levels, making this agent particularly suitable for the treatment of oral infection (Force and Nahata 1995). The use of miconazole oral gel was effective in the treatment of acute candidiasis caused by the use of topical intranasal steroids (Kyrmizakis et al. 1999).

Unfortunately, in recent years, the prevalence of resistance to conventional antifungal drugs increased considerably (Redding et al. 2000). This resistance may be resultant of several mechanisms (White et al. 2002), including increased production of lanosterol demethylase. Changes in the demethylase enzyme structure make the cell less susceptible to the action of the azole.

Additionally, the successful treatment of candidiasis may be impaired where there is an established biofilm. Biofilms exhibit significantly greater tolerance to traditional antifungals (Ramage et al. 2002). As this form is frequently found in oral milieu, this is an additional challenge in the treatment of oral infections.

Alternative strategies have been suggested to the treatment of oral fungal infections, including modification of biomaterials to inhibit *Candida* adhesion (Chandra et al. 2005; Price et al. 2005; Redding et al. 2009). Quaternary ammonium silane-functionalized methacrylate (QAMS) is synthesized macromonomer with activity against *Candida albicans* biofilms (Gong et al. 2012). Also, incorporation of silver nanoparticles in denture base acrylic showed good antimicrobial activity (Nam et al. 2012). Other strategies explore the quorum-sensing process, promoting breakdown of farnesol in biofilm, resulting in considerable instability. Another possible strategy involves the use of locally administered probiotics (Van der Mei et al. 2000; Meurman 2005; Hatakka et al. 2007) (mixture of *Bifidobacterium longum, Lactobacillus bulgaricus,* and *Streptococcus thermophiles*), which improved clinical conditions and reduced candidal prevalence (Li et al. 2013).

References

Adebola AR, Adeleke SI, Mukhtar M, Osunde OD, Akhiwu BI, Ladeinde A (2012) Oral manifestation of HIV/AIDS infections in paediatric Nigerian patients. Niger Med J 53(3):150–154

Al-Mohaya MA, Darwazeh AM, Bin-Salih S, Al-Khudair W (2009) Oral lesions in Saudi renal transplant patients. Saudi J Kidney Dis Transpl 20(1):20–29

Andes D (2003) In vivo pharmacodynamics of antifungal drugs in treatment of candidiasis. Antimicrob Agents Chemother 47:1179–1186

Bodhade AS, Ganvir SM, Hazarey VK (2011) Oral manifestations of HIV infection and their correlation with CD4 count. J Oral Sci 53(2):203–211

Ceballos-Salobreña A, Gaitaín-Cepeda L, Ceballos-García L, Samaranayake LP (2004) The effect of antiretroviral therapy on the prevalence of HIV-associated oral candidiasis in a Spanish cohort. Oral Surg Oral Med Oral Pathol Oral Radiol Endod 97(3):345–350

Chandra J, Patel JD, Li J, Zhou G, Mukherjee PK, McCormick TS et al (2005) Modification of surface properties of biomaterials influences the ability of *Candida albicans* to form biofilms. Appl Environ Microbiol 71:8795–8801

Ellepola AN, Samaranayake LP (2000) Oral candida infections and antimycotics. Crit Rev Oral Biol Med 11:172–198

Ellepola AN, Samaranayake LP (2001) Inhalational and topical steroids and oral candidosis: a mini review. Oral Dis 7:211–216

Farah CS, Ashman RB, Challacombe SJ (2000) Oral candidosis. Clin Dermatol 18:553–562

Farah CS, Lynch N, McCullough MJ (2010) Oral fungal infections: an update for the general practitioner. Aust Dent J 55(1 Suppl):48–54

Fine DH (1988) Mouth rinses as adjuncts for plaque and gingivitis management. A status report for the American Journal of Dentistry. Am J Dent 1:259–263

Force RW, Nahata MC (1995) Salivary concentrations of ketoconazole and fluconazole: implications for drug efficacy in oropharyngeal and esophageal candidiasis. Ann Pharmacother 29:10–15

Gaitan Cepeda LA, Ceballos Salobreña A, López Ortega K, Arzate Mora N, Jiménez SY (2008) Oral lesions and immune reconstitution syndrome in HIV+/AIDS patients receiving highly active antiretroviral therapy. Epidemiological evidence. Med Oral Patol Oral Cir Bucal 13(2):E85–E93

Gaurav S, Keerthilatha PM, Archna N (2011) Prevalence of oral manifestations and their association with CD4/CD8 Ratio and HIV viral load in South India. Int J Dent 2011:964278

Giannini PJ, Shetty KV (2011) Diagnosis and management of oral candidiasis. Otolaryngol Clin North Am 44:231–240

Gonçalves LS, Júnior AS, Ferreira SM, Sousa CO, Fontes TV, Vettore MV, Torres SR (2013) Factors associated with specific clinical forms of oral candidiasis in HIV-infected Brazilian adults. Arch Oral Biol 58(6):657–663

Gong SQ, Niu LN, Kemp LK, Yiu CK, Ryou H, Qi YP, Blizzard JD, Nikonov S, Brackett MG, Messer RL, Wu CD, Mao J, Bryan Brister L, Rueggeberg FA, Arola DD, Pashley DH, Tay FR (2012) Quaternary ammonium silane-functionalized, methacrylate resin composition with antimicrobial activities and self-repair potential. Acta Biomater 8(9):3270–3282. doi:10.1016/j.actbio.2012.05.031, Epub 2012 May 29

Gonsalves WC, Wrightson AS, Henry RG (2008) Common oral conditions in older persons. Am Fam Physician 78(7):845–852

Hatakka K, Ahola AJ, Yli-Knuuttila H, Richardson M, Poussa T, Meurman JH et al (2007) Probiotics reduce the prevalence of oral Candida in the elderly a randomized controlled trial. J Dent Res 86:125–130

Krishnan PA (2012) Fungal infections of the oral mucosa. Indian J Dent Res 23(5):650–659

Kyrmizakis DE, Papadakis CE, Lohuis PJ, Manolarakis G, Karakostas E, Amanakis Z (1999) Acute candidiasis of the oro- and hypopharynx as the result of topical intranasal steroids administration. Rhinology 38(2):87–89

Lalla RV, Patton LL, Dongari-Bagtzoglou A (2013) Oral candidiasis: pathogenesis, clinical presentation, diagnosis and treatment strategies. J Calif Dent Assoc 41(4):263–268

Li D, Li Q, Liu C, Lin M, Li X, Xiao X, Zhu Z, Gong Q, Zhou H (2013) Efficacy and safety of probiotics in the treatment of Candida-associated stomatitis. Mycoses. doi: 10.1111/myc.12116. [Epub ahead of print]

Lourenço AG, Motta AC, Figueiredo LT, Machado AA, Komesu MC (2011) Oral lesions associated with HIV infection before and during the antiretroviral therapy era in Ribeirão Preto. Brazil J Oral Sci 53(3):379–385

Meurman JH (2005) Probiotics: do they have a role in oral medicine and dentistry? Eur J Oral Sci 113:188–196

Nam KY, Lee CH, Lee CJ (2012) Antifungal and physical characteristics of modified denture base acrylic incorporated with silver nanoparticles. Gerodontology 29(2):e413–e419

Neville BW, Damm DD, Allen CM, Bouquot JE (2009) Fungal and protozoal diseases. In: Neville BW, Damm DD, Allen CM (eds) Bouquot oral and maxillofacial pathology, 3rd edn. W.B. Saunder, Philadelphia, pp 224–237

Nimmi M, Firth NA, Cannon RD (2010) Antifungal drug resistance of oral fungi. Odontology 98:15–25

Okamoto MR, Kamoi M, Yamachika S, Tsurumoto A, Imamura T, Yamamoto K, Kadomatsu S, Saito I, Maeda N, Nakagawa Y (2013) Efficacy of Fungiflora Y staining for the diagnosis of oral erythematous candidiasis. Gerodontology 30(3):220–225

Price CL, Williams DW, Waters MG, Coulthwaite L, Verran J, Taylor RL et al (2005) Reduced adherence of Candida to silane treated silicone rubber. J Biomed Mater Res B Appl Biomater 74:481–487

Pusateri CR, Monaco EA, Edgerton M (2009) Sensitivity of *Candida albicans* biofilm cells grown on denture acrylic to antifungal proteins and chlorhexidine. Arch Oral Biol 54:588–594

Ramage G, VandeWalle K, Bachmann SP, Wickes BL, Lopez-Ribot JL (2002) In vitro pharmacodynamic properties of three antifungal agents against preformed *Candida albicans* biofilms determined by time-kill studies. Antimicrob Agents Chemother 46:3634–3636

Ramage G, Jose A, Coco B, Rajendran R, Rautemaa R, Murray C, Lappin DF, Bagg J (2011) Commercial mouthwashes are more effective than azole antifungals against *Candida albicans* biofilms in vitro. Oral Surg Oral Med Oral Pathol Oral Radiol Endod 111(4):456–460

Redding SW, Kirkpatrick WR, Dib O, Fothergill AW, Rinaldi MG, Patterson TF (2000) The epidemiology of non-albicans Candida in oropharyngeal candidiasis in HIV patients. Spec Care Dentist 20:178–181

Redding S, Bhatt B, Rawls HR, Siegel G, Scott K, Lopez-Ribot J (2009) Inhibition of Candida albicans biofilm formation on denture material. Oral Surg Oral Med Oral Pathol Oral Radiol Endod 107:669–672

Samaranayake L (2006) Essential microbiology for dentistry, 3rd edn. Churchill Livingstone, Edinburgh, p 255, 62–64

Sanglard D, Bille J (2002) Current understanding of the modes of action of and resistance mechanisms to conventional and emerging antifungal agents for treatment of Candida infections. In: Calderone RA (ed) *Candida* and candidiasis. ASM Press, Washington, DC, pp 349–383

Scully C (2004) Candidiasis. In: Scully C (ed) Oral and maxillofacial medicine. Elsevier, London, pp 252–269

Sharma G, Pai KM, Suhas S, Ramapuram JT, Doshi D, Anup N (2006) Oral manifestations in HIV/AIDS infected patients from India. Oral Dis 12(6): 537–542

Soysa NS, Samaranayake LP, Ellepola AN (2008) Antimicrobials as a contributory factor in oral candidosis – a brief overview. Oral Dis 14:138–143

Terai H, Shimahara M (2009) Usefulness of culture test and direct examination for the diagnosis of oral atrophic candidiasis. Int J Dermatol 48:371–373

Thorman R, Neovius M, Hylander B (2009) Prevalence and early detection of oral fungal infection: a cross-sectional controlled study in a group of Swedish end-stage renal disease patients. Scand J Urol Nephrol 43(4):325–330

Tirwomwe JF, Rwenyonyi CM, Muwazi LM, Besigye B, Mboli F (2007) Oral manifestations of HIV/AIDS in clients attending TASO clinics in Uganda. Clin Oral Investig 11(3):289–292

Van der Mei HC, Free RH, Elving GJ, Van Weissenbruch R, Albers FW, Busscher HJ (2000) Effect of probiotic bacteria on prevalence of yeasts in oropharyngeal biofilms on silicone rubber voice prostheses in vitro. J Med Microbiol 49:713–718

White TC, Holleman S, Dy F, Mirels LF, Stevens DA (2002) Resistance mechanisms in clinical isolates of *Candida albicans*. Antimicrob Agents Chemother 46:1704–1713

Williams DW, Lewis MA (2000) Isolation and identification of *Candida* from the oral cavity. Oral Dis 6:3–11

Williams DW, Kuriyama T, Silva S, Malic S, Lewis MAO (2011) *Candida* biofilms and oral candidosis: treatment and prevention. Periodontology 2000 55:250–265

Worthington HV, Clarkson JE, Eden OB (2007) Interventions for treating oral candidiasis for patients with cancer receiving treatment. Cochrane Database Syst Rev 2, CD001972

Acute and Chronic Pseudomembranous Candidosis

6

Paulo Henrique Couto Souza
and Soraya de A. Berti Couto

Abstract

Candidosis is a common opportunistic fungal infection caused by several Candida species and *Candida albicans* is often associated with oral infections. It has been described as an important disease that affected the oral cavity of a significant population percentage. Oral candidosis may present several clinical types and the pseudomembranous or "thrush", as is popularly known, is one of the most recognized. According to some authors, pseudomembranous candidosis can be classified as acute or chronic infection. The objective of this chapter is to present important and current data regarding the epidemiology, etiology, clinical characteristics, diagnostic criteria, and biological behavior of acute and chronic pseudomembranous candidosis.

Candidosis is a common opportunistic fungal infection caused by several Candida species and *Candida albicans* is often associated with oral infections (Akpan and Morgan 2002; Farah et al., 2010; Muzyka 2005). It has been described as an important disease that affected the oral cavity of a significant population percentage (Chandrasekar and Molinari 1985; Shepherd 1986). Oral Candidosis may present several clinical types and the pseudomembranous or "thrush", as is popularly known, is one of the most recognized (Neville et al., 2004). This type of oral Candidosis was firstly described by the French pediatrician Francois Valleix in 1838 (Kumar and Alexander 2013).

According to some authors, pseudomembranous Candidosis can be classified as acute or chronic infection (Muzyka and Epifanio 2013; Neville et al., 2004). The acute infection is a peculiar clinical manifestation of this opportunistic fungal disease, taking into account its rapid oral manifestation usually related to broad-spectrum antibiotic exposure, which disrupts the balance in the oral microbiota (Eversole et al., 2012; Neville et al., 2004). Clinically, it can appear as white or yellow plaques on any mucosal surface; however, the lesions appear more frequently on the buccal mucosa, soft palate, tongue,

P.H.C. Souza (✉) • S.de.A. Berti Couto
Stomatology, School of Health and Biosciences,
Pontifícia Universidade Católica do Paraná,
Curitiba, Brazil
e-mail: couto.s@pucpr.br

E.A.R. Rosa (ed.), *Oral Candidosis: Physiopathology, Decision Making, and Therapeutics*,
DOI 10.1007/978-3-662-47194-4_6

and lips (Laskaris 2004). The plaques represent an overgrowth of the yeast on the mucosa, leading to epithelial cell desquamation and a concomitant accumulation of bacteria, keratin, and necrotic tissue (Kumar and Alexander 2013). Chronic infection usually stays for a longer period than acute and may be present in immunocompromised patients as those transplanted, affected by HIV, leukemia (Akpan and Morgan 2002), endocrine disorders (Epstein et al., 2002; Muzyka 2005; Neville et al., 2004), and in those submitted to systemic corticosteroid use, chemo- and radiotherapy (Farah et al., 2000; Gonsalves et al. 2007; Little et al. 2008). The objective of this chapter is to present important and current data regarding the epidemiology, etiology, clinical characteristics, diagnostic criteria, and biological behavior of acute and chronic pseudomembranous candidosis.

Epidemiology

Candidosis is the most common oral fungal infection diagnosed in humans, especially in earlier and later periods of life (Akpan and Morgan 2002; Muzyka 2005; Neville et al., 2004). The incidence of pseudomembranous candidosis, including both patterns, acute and chronic, varies according to the population studied and depends on the presence of some risk factors (Akpan and Morgan 2002; Farah et al., 2000). Among these, the pathogen (*Candida species* strains), immune status of the host, and the presence of local and systemic factors can be highlighted (Akpan and Morgan 2002; Farah et al., 2000; Neville et al., 2004). The local and systemic factors include wearing dentures, impaired salivary gland function, endocrine disorders as diabetes mellitus, immunologic disorders as HIV, chemo- and radiotherapy, drug therapy as corticosteroid, immunomodulatory, cytotoxic and xerostomic drugs, besides nutritional factors (Akpan and Morgan 2002; Farah et al., 2000, 2010; Gonsalves et al., 2007). In addition, this form of candidosis is common amongst patients who are immunocompromised, in particular those taking antimitotic drugs and/or corticosteroids and also those patients with HIV infection (McCullough and Savage 2005). Besides, some authors have reported a higher prevalence of acute pseudomembranous in kidney transplant patients (Sahebjamee et al., 2010).

There is no prevalence by sex or age in Candidosis (Scully 2009). However, some studies have reported that this infection could affect especially newborns, infants, and elderly people (Akpan and Morgan 2002; Gonsalves et al., 2007; Muzyka 2005). In newborns and infants, the infection is usually superficial and easy to manage, mainly when in these patients the acute pseudomembranous Candidosis occurs as an opportunistic and transitory infection predisposed by their undeveloped immune system (McCullough and Savage 2005; Neville et al., 2004). However, oral Candidosis among preterm or hospitalized critically ill infants can, rarely, become systemic and potentially fatal (Shetty et al., 2005). On the other side, in elderly persons, the most readily recognized clinical pattern, acute pseudomembranous Candidosis, is characterized by adherent, curd-like plaques that can be removed by wiping firmly with a tongue blade or gauze (Gonsalves et al., 2008). Besides, Gonsalves et al. (2007) and Gonsalves et al. (2008) referred that Candidosis is one of the most frequent oral diseases in older persons. It is estimated that the frequency of the Candidosis varies around 5 % in neonates, 5 % in patients with cancer, and in 10 % of the elderly, debilitated, or hospitalized patients. In addition, this infection is common in more than half of patients undergoing chemo- and/or radiotherapy (Davies et al., 2008; Regezi and Sciubba 2008; Soysa et al., 2004). Glaber et al. (2008) evaluated the incidence of oral candidosis in hospitalized patients who had HIV and the result showed that 50.7 % of the patients had oral candidosis and the pseudomembranous form was found to be most frequent.

Etiology and Etiopathogenesis

The most common fungi associated with the pseudomembranous candidosis etiology is *Candida albicans*. The genus Candida is characterized as including white asporogenous (imperfect) yeasts capable of forming pseudohyphae. Within the genus, species are characterized primarily on colonial morphology, carbon utilization, and fermentation. There are seven *Candida species* of major medical importance and the most important of these is *C. albicans*, which is isolated most frequently (over 80 %) and it is considered to be the more virulent in humans (McCullough et al., 1999). Yet, the non-albicans *Candida spp.* are also implicated in the etiology of oral Candidosis and in those cases, they may have significant implications for the general health of immunosuppressed patients (McIntyre 2001). Amongst the non-albicans types, *C. tropicalis*, *C. glabrata*, *C. parapsilosis*, *C. stellatoidea*, *C. krusei* and *C. kefyr*, and more recently, *C. dubliniensis* in immunocompromised patients, have been associated as etiology agents of oral Candidosis (Al-Karaawi et al., 2002; Farah et al., 2010; McCullough et al., 1996). Epstein (1990) referred that some species such as *C. glabrata* and *C. tropicalis* account for approximately 5–8 % of oral isolates, respectively. In newborns, the *C. parapsilosis* is frequently found (Scully 2009).

Antibiotic Therapy × Acute Pseudomembranous Candidosis

One of the important predisposing factors for the acute form of pseudomembranous Candidosis is the antibiotic therapy (Neville et al., 2004). In this context, some studies have reported that besides the classical manifestation of this infection in infants, which is the acute pseudomembranous candidosis, there would be a second manifestation of oral Candidosis called the oropharyngeal Candidosis form, as a side effect of antibiotic treatment in these patients, especially when penicillins and the association of clavulanate—amoxicillin were prescribed (Tres and Urtiaga 2001). In the same way, there was a strong relation between oral Candidosis and newborns when they were hospitalized in neonatal intensive care unit (NICU) under prolonged antibiotic therapy and the acute pseudomembranous Candidosis was the most common presentation (Gupta et al., 1996). In these patients, *Candida albicans* was isolated in 50 % cases, besides *C. tropicalis*, *C. paratropicalis*, *C. krusei*, *C. glabrata*, and *C. parapsilosis*. In addition, the use of broad-spectrum antibiotics may predispose patients to alterations in commensal oral microbiota. In healthy persons, oral microbiota influences candida levels through competition for dietary substrates and epithelial cell adhesion. Thus, alterations in commensal microbiota may result in Candida overgrowth (Farah et al., 2000, 2010; Soysa et al., 2008).

Predisposing Factors × Chronic Pseudomembranous Candidosis

The main difference between acute and chronic pseudomembranous Candidosis is the duration of the infection. The latter is present for a longer period when compare to the former one. Usually, the infection occurs due to, at least, three main characteristics: immune status of the patient, oral mucosal environment, and also resistance strain of *Candida albicans* (Neville et al., 2004). It is important to state that some predisposing factors can be associated to the occurrence of the chronic form of the Candidosis as endocrine disorders (Epstein et al., 2002; Muzyka 2005; Neville et al., 2004), Sjogren's Syndrome (Neville et al., 2004), patients who presented immunocompromised like that affected by leukemia, HIV and transplanted (Akpan and Morgan 2002; Soames and Southam 2008) and in those patients who received some kinds of medications as inhaled or systemic corticosteroid for a long time (Farah et al., 2000; Gonsalves et al., 2007; Little et al., 2008; Muzyka 2005). Patients undergoing antineoplastic treatment (radio and/or chemotherapy) are likely to develop opportunistic infections such as oral candidosis (Little et al., 2008).

In the most part of the predisposing factors previously cited, *Candida albicans* can infect the oral cavity secondarily due to the reduction in salivary flow and also because of changes in the saliva composition (Little et al., 2008). The reduction of salivary flow compromises the function of some important enzymes in the saliva as lactoferrin, sialoperoxidase and lysozyme, which are responsible for the maintenance of oral homeostasis. Furthermore, salivary flow serves to dilute and remove potential pathogenic organisms from the oral mucosa (Muzyka 2005).

There are a lot of medications that decrease salivary output and consequently may favor the occurrence of candidosis (Muzyka 2005). Among these medications, we can highlight antihistamines, antidepressants, antihypertensives, decongestants agents, antipsychotics, anxyolitics, and sedatives (Neville et al., 2004). Muzyka (2005) referred that the inhaled corticosteroids used to treat airway inflammation of bronchial asthma has presented good results and can reduce or even eliminate the systemic use of these medications. However, inhaled corticosteroids have been associated with an increased risk for oral candidosis (Alsaeedi 2002).

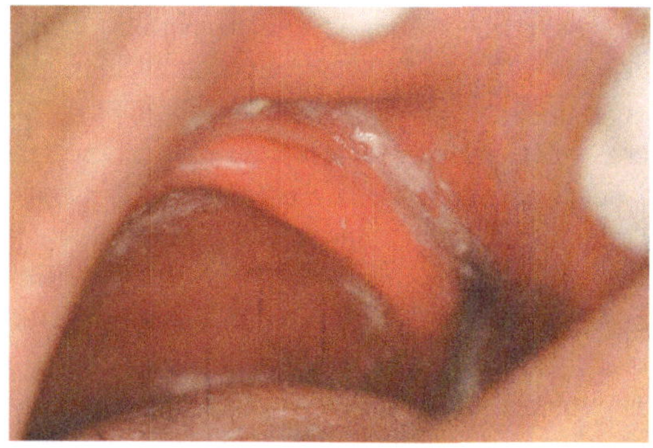

Fig. 6.1 Chronic pseudomembranous candidosis located in left upper deep bucal vestibule and hard palate in a patient submitted to the chemotherapy

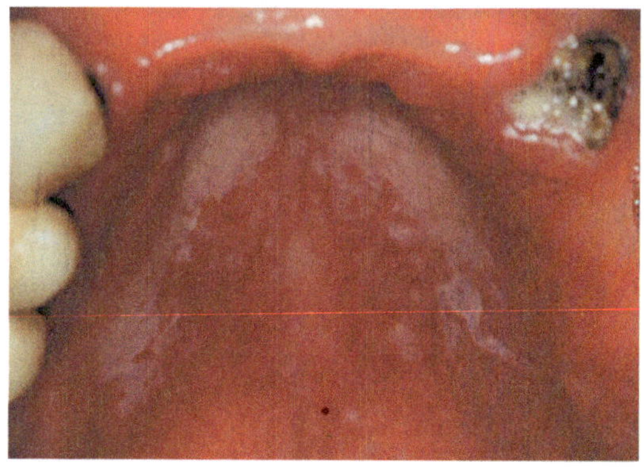

Fig. 6.2 Chronic pseudomembranous candidosis located in hard palate in a patient with an uncontrolled diabetes mellitus

Clinical Characteristics

Clinically, pseudomembranous candidosis is characterized by the presence of adherent white or yellow plaques located on any oral mucosa surface (Farah et al., 2000; Gonsalves et al., 2008; Muzyka 2005), which can resemble buttermilk (Samaranayake et al., 2000), and size can vary from small plates until confluent areas affecting multiples sites (Figs. 6.1 and 6.2). The plaques can be removed by rubbing the mucosa affected with a gauze (Farah et al., 2000; Gonsalves et al., 2008; Muzyka 2005). After removing plaque, the underlying mucosa may present erythematous and/or bleeding (Neville et al., 2004; Samaranayake et al., 2000).

The lesions are usually asymptomatic (Farah et al., 2010; Gonsalves et al., 2008); however, some patients can refer burning sensation, unpleasant salty or bitter taste (Gonsalves et al., 2008; Muzyka 2005; Neville et al., 2004; Regezi and Sciubba 2008). According to Muzyka (2005), these symptoms may compromise chewing and swallowing.

Pseudomembranous candidosis can be located in several anatomic sites of the oral mucosa surface, but the preference localization included mucosa of checks, deep buccal vestibule, oropharynx, and tongue (Farah et al., 2000; McCullough and Savage 2005; Neville et al., 2004). Gabler et al. (2008)) have identified that the main anatomic localization of the pseudomembranous candidosis in HIV patients were tongue (55.5 %), buccal mucosa (37 %), and palate (7.4 %).

Diagnosis

Candidosis diagnosis usually can be made according to the clinical findings (Muzyka 2005).

Basically, both acute and chronic pseudomembranous Candidosis are diagnosed by the white plaques removal using a soaked gauze or a wood spatula. Normally, after the removal, it is possible to see an underlying mucosa showing an erythematous surface. In advanced cases, the full oral mucosa can be affected (Shaffer et al., 1987). However, some authors state that the diagnosis of acute pseudomembranous candidosis has been overestimated during the last years and for this reason, in immunocompromised patients, a smear stained for Gram should be carried out to the differential diagnosis of acute pseudomembranous candidosis with yellow or white plaques caused by opportunistic bacteria (Scully 2009). Mostly, the associated symptoms are minimal, yet, in severe cases, the patients may complain of sensibility, burning, and dysphagia. Interestingly, some authors have described that the persistence of pseudomembranous candidosis can result in loss of pseudomembrane, with the presentation of a red lesion more generally known as acute erythematous candidosis. In these cases, along the dorsum of the tongue, it is possible to observe areas of depapillation and dekeratinization (Regezi and Sciubba 2008).

However, it is also important to highlight the patient's history and the response to treatment with antifungal drugs (Gonsalves et al., 2008). In addition to the clinical findings, the diagnosis can be confirmed with exfoliative cytology, swab culture, imprint culture and, in specific cases, with mucosal biopsy (Gonsalves et al., 2008; Muzyka 2005). The exfoliative cytology is able to differentiate yeast and hyphal forms of the fungal, but is less sensitive than culture methods (Williams and Lewis 2000). Swab culture is the technique used to identify the microorganism and consists in obtaining a specimen by scraping the surface of the lesion using a swab. This specimen is deposited on a specific culture medium and incubated. *Candida albicans* grows after 2–3 days of incubation (Neville et al., 2004).

Exfoliative cytology, swab cultures, and biopsy are generally used to verify, qualitatively, the presence of different *Candida species*; however, these methods are less sensitive than culture. Imprint culture and salivary rinse techniques are able to quantify *Candida species*, and furthermore differentiate normal levels of *Candida spp.*, those considered pathological, which are responsible for disease onset (Muzyka 2005).

Dendritic Cells × *Candida albicans*

The strategic location of dendritic cells in tissues, specifically in the epidermis and mucous membranes suggests that these cells assume a primary role in the onset of immune response against microorganisms such as Candida (Newman and Holly 2001). In addition, dendritic cells act differently on *Candida albicans*. For example, immature myeloid dendritic cells, phagocytose the fungus in both forms, effectively and quickly. However, those ones that remain in the filament or tubular form, known as "hypha", are able to "escape" from the phagosomes. This occurs by different mechanisms of phagocytosis. When the microorganism is phagocytosed in its unicellular form, known as "yeast", the fungus is surrounded by pseudopodia throughout its surface up to be fully enclosed, following the formation of the phagosome in which different stages of cell degradation is observed over a period of 4 h. However, in its hypha form, the fungus is engaged bilaterally by the emission of pseudopodia until its encapsulation, followed by the formation of the phagosome in which, surprisingly, within one hour, Candida seems to break the membrane of the phagosome, remaining free in the cell cytoplasm (d'Ostiani et al., 2000). Furthermore, the host resistance in candidosis is the result of Th1-mediated response along with the synthesis of cytokines such as IFN- and IL-12 γ, since they induce phagocytosis. Nevertheless, the response mediated by Th2 lymphocytes and their cytokines such as IL -4 and IL -10, inhibit Th1 development and inactivate cellular phagocytosis mechanism, allowing the disease progression (Bacci et al., 2002). Then, once taking the form of unicellular yeast, the Candida fungus induces dendritic cells to produce IL-12 cytokine, which in turn draws the Th1 lymphocytes, which are important in resistance to antigen in question. In contrast with in the tubular or filamentous form, the fungus induces dendritic cells to produce cytokine IL-4 by attracting Th2 lymphocytes, which act to inactivate the process of phagocytosis of Candida, as mentioned by Torosantucci et al. (2004).

References

Akpan A, Morgan R (2002) Oral candidiasis. Postgrad Med J 78:455–459

Al-Karaawi ZM, Manfredi M, Waugh AC, McCullough MJ, Jorge J, Scully C, Porter SR (2002) Molecular characterization of Candida spp. isolated from the oral cavities of patients from diverse clinical settings. Oral Microbiol Immunol 17:44–49

Alsaeedi A (2002) The effects of inhaled corticosteroids in chronic obstructive pulmonary disease: a systematic review of randomized placebo-controlled trials. Am J Med 113(1):59–65

Bacci A, Montagnoli C, Perruccio K, Bozza S, Gaziano R, Pitzurra L, Velardi A, d'Ostiani CF, Cutler JE, Romani L (2002) Dendritic cells pulsed with fungal RNA induce protective immunity to Candida albicans in hematopoietic transplantation. J Immunol 168(6):2904–2913

Chandrasekar PH, Molinari JA (1985) Oral candidosis: forerunner of acquired immunodeficiency syndrome? Oral Surg Oral Med Oral Pathol 60:532–534

Davies AN, Brailsford SR, Beighton D, Shorthose K, Stevens VC (2008) Oral candidosis in community-based patients with advanced cancer. J Pain Symptom Manage 35(5):508–514

d'Ostiani CF, Del Sero G, Bacci A, Montagnoli C, Spreca A, Mencacci A, Ricciardi-Castagnoli P, Romani L (2000) Dendritic cells discriminate between yeasts and hyphae of the fungus Candida albicans: implications for initiation of T helper cell immunity in vitro and in vivo. J Exp Med 191(10):1661–1674

Epstein JB (1990) Antifungal therapy in oropharyngeal mycotic infections. Oral Surg Oral Med Oral Pathol 69(1):32–41

Epstein JB, Gorsky M, Caldwell J (2002) Fluconazole mouthrinses for oral candidiasis in postirradiation, transplant, and other patients. Oral Surg Oral Med Oral Pathol Oral Radiol Endod 93(6):671–675

Eversole LR, Wysocki GP, Sapp JP (2012) Patologia Bucomaxilofacial Contemporânea, 2ª Ed. Editora Santos, 464p

Farah CS, Ashman RB, Challacombe SJ (2000) Oral candidosis. Clin Dermatol 18(5):553–562

Farah CS, Lynch N, McCullough MJ (2010) Oral fungal infections: an update for the general practitioner. Aust Dent J 55(Suppl 1):48–54

Gabler IG, Barbosa AC, Vilela RR, Lyon S, Rosa CA (2008) Incidence and anatomic localization of oral candidiasis in patients with aids hospitalized in a public hospital in Belo Horizonte, MG. Brazil J Appl Oral Sci 16(4):247–250

Gonsalves WC, Chi AA, Neville BW (2007) Common oral lesions: Part I. Superficial mucosal lesions. Am Fam Physician 75:501–507

Gonsalves WC, Wrightson AS, Henry RG (2008) Common oral conditions in older persons. Am Fam Physician 78(1):846–852

Gupta P, Faridi MM, Rawat S, Sharma P (1996) Clinical profile and risk factors for oral candidosis in sick newborns. Indian Pediatr 33(4):299–303

Kumar M, Alexander P (2013) Thrush. eMedicine [serial on the Internet]. http:// www.emedicine.com/ped/topic2245.htm#section$miscellaneous. Accessed 25 Sept 2013

Laskaris G (2004) Atlas Colorido de Doenças da Boca, 3ª Ed. Artmed, 454p

Little JW, Falace DA, Miller CS, Rhodus NL (2008) Manejo odontológico do paciente clinicamente comprometido, 7ª Ed. Elsevier Editora Ltda

McCullough MJ, Savage NW (2005) Oral candidosis and the therapeutic use of antifungal agents in dentistry. Aust Dent J 50(Suppl 2):S36–S39

McCullough MJ, Ross BC, Reade PC (1996) Candida albicans: a review of its history, taxonomy, epidemiology, virulence attributes, and methods of strain differentiation. Int J Oral Maxillofac Surg 25:136–144

McCullough MJ, Clemons KV, Stevens DA (1999) Molecular epidemiology of the global and temporal diversity of Candida albicans. Clin Infect Dis 29(5):1220–1225

McIntyre GT (2001) Oral candidosis. Dent Update 28(3):132–139

Muzyka BC (2005) Oral fungal infections. Dent Clin N Am 49:49–65

Muzyka BC, Epifanio RN (2013) Update on oral fungal infections. Dent Clin N Am 57:561–581

Neville BW, Damm DD, Allen CM, Bouquot JE (2004) Patologia Oral e Maxilofacial, 3ª Ed. Elsevier Editora Ltda

Newman SL, Holly A (2001) Candida albicans is phagocytosed, killed, and processed for antigen presentation by human dendritic cells. Infect Immun 69(11):6813–6822

Regezi JA, Sciubba JJ (2008) Patologia Bucal: Correlações Clínico-Patológicas, 5ª Ed. Elsevier Editora Ltda, 417p

Sahebjamee M, Shakur SM, Nikoobakht MR, Momen BJ, Mansourian A (2010) Oral lesions in kidney transplant patients. Iran J Kidney Dis 4(3):232–236

Samaranayake LP, Leung WK, Jin L (2000) Oral mucosal fungal infections. Periodontol 49:39–59

Scully C (2009) Medicina Oral e Maxilofacial – Bases do Diagnóstico e Tratamento, 2ª Ed. Elsevier Editora Ltda., 408 p

Shaffer WG, Hine MK, Levy BM (1987) Tratado de Patologia Bucal, 4ª ed. Guanabara Koogan, Rio de Janeiro, 837p

Shepherd MG (1986) The pathogenesis and host defense mechanisms of oral candidosis. N Z Dent J 2:78–81

Shetty SS, Harrison LH, Hajjeh RA, Taylor T, Mirza SA, Schmidt AB, Sanza LT, Shutt KA, Fridkin SK (2005)

Determining risk factors for candidemia among newborn infants from population-based surveillance. Pediatr Infect Dis J 24(7):601–604

Soames JV, Southam JC (2008) Patologia Oral, 4th Ed. Editora Guanabara

Soysa NI, Samaranayake LP, Ellepola ANB (2004) Cytotoxic drugs, radiotherapy and oral candidiasis. Oral Oncol 40:971–978

Soysa NS, Samaranayake LP, Ellepola AN (2008) Antimicrobials as a contributory factor in oral candidosis – a brief overview. Oral Dis 14(2):138–143

Torosantucci A, Romagnoli G, Chiani P, Stringaro A, Crateri P, Mariotti S, Teloni R, Arancia G, Cassone A, Nisini R (2004) Candida albicans yeast and germ tube forms interfere differently with human monocyte differentiation into dendritic cells: a novel dimorphism-dependent mechanism to escape the host's immune response. Infect Immun 72(2):833–843

Tres JC, Urtiaga M (2001) Candidiasis secondary to antibiotic treatment in primary care. An Sist Sanit Navar 24(3):283–299

Williams DW, Lewis MA (2000) Isolation and identification of Candida from the oral cavity. Oral Dis 6(1):3–11

Candida-Associated Denture Stomatitis: Clinical Relevant Aspects

7

Andréa Araújo de Vasconcellos,
Letícia Machado Gonçalves, Altair A. Del Bel Cury,
and Wander José da Silva

Abstract

Candida-associated denture stomatitis is a common fungal infection that affects removable denture wearers. Although *Candida* spp. are considered commensal fungal in the oral cavity, changes in local and/or systemic predisposing factors related to the host conditions may lead to pathogenic form and cause disease. The clinical manifestations are usually associated with the predisposing factors, changing from no symptoms to severe pain and difficulty swallowing. The therapeutic strategies commonly adopted in the clinical practice are the use of topical and/or systemic antifungal, in addition to removing mechanically the plaque from denture surfaces and from underlying mucosa and give instructions about the correct oral hygiene to the patient. In this context, considering the high prevalence of this disease in the clinical practice, a review about the etiology, risk factors, clinical manifestations, and therapy management of these patients is of utmost importance.

Introduction

Candida-associated denture stomatitis is a predominantly fungal infection that affects the human oral cavity (Harriott and Noverr 2011). Although *Candida* spp. may be involved during infection, *Candida albicans* are considered the main pathogens, and have been found in a commensalism form in the oral cavities of adults and children, without any clinical disease (Lalla et al., 2013). These microorganisms are encountered in the dentition, tongue, cheeks, palatal mucosa, restorative materials, and oral protheses (Sánchez-Vargas et al., 2013).

A.A. de Vasconcellos
Faculty of Dentistry, Federal University of Ceará, Sobral, Ceará, Brazil

L.M. Gonçalves
Faculty of Dentistry, CEUMA University, São Luiz do Maranhão, Maranhão, Brazil

A.A. Del Bel Cury • W.J. da Silva (✉)
Department of Prosthodontics and Periodontology, Piracicaba Dental School, State University of Campinas, Piracicaba, SP, Brazil
e-mail: wanderjose@fop.unicamp.br

E.A.R. Rosa (ed.), *Oral Candidosis: Physiopathology, Decision Making, and Therapeutics*,
DOI 10.1007/978-3-662-47194-4_7

However, local and/or systemic predisposition factors may lead commensal microorganisms to pathogenic form, providing an oral environment adequate to the adhesion of microorganisms to the denture surface and mucosal epithelial cells (Sardi et al., 2013). This is followed by cell multiplication, organization, and secretion of extracellular matrix, resulting in the formation of biofilm, an highly organized three-dimensional structure (Jayatilake 2011).

Also, *C. albicans* may be found in two major forms, yeast and hyphae form. The yeast form is usually associated with mucosal commensalism, although the conversion yeast-to-hyphae is commonly related to the invasion of superficial layers of the oral epithelium, leading to clinical infection (Vallejo et al., 2013).

Epidemiology

Although *Candida albicans* have been the main pathogens of CADS, *C. glabrata*, *C. Tropicalis*, and *C. parapsilosis* has been found less frequently (Vazquez and Sobel 2002; Dorocka-Bobkowska and Konopka 2007). Some factors favor the development of *C. albicans* biofilms, such as its capability to stick and proliferate through the denture surfaces and oral mucosal epithelial and produce a complex and heterogeneous bacterial biofilm (Salerno et al., 2011).

CADS has been found in 60–65 % of the denture wearers with more diffused clinical manifestations, but considering the patients that do not manifest clinical signs of inflammation and infection, this percentage increases to 75 % (Salerno et al., 2011; Webb et al., 1998a). It was reported that CADS is the most common oral mucosal lesion associated with removable dentures (Cueto et al., 2013), and affects one in every three complete denture wearers (Zissis et al., 2006).

Risk Factors

The changes from commensal to pathogenic form of *Candida* spp. are typically caused by local and/or systemic predisposing factors related to the host conditions, favoring the development of the disease. While the local factors provide an adequate oral environment to biofilm development, the systemic factors influence the defense host mechanisms (Lalla et al., 2013; Salerno et al., 2011).

Local Factors

The local factors are important to favor the biofilm accumulation in the oral environment. In this context, different factors such as irradiation, trauma, xerostomy, complete denture wearers, poor dental hygiene, smoke, carbohydrate-rich diet, and environmental pH will be discussed.

The irradiation is considered a risk factor, considering that it leads to hiposalivation (Nett et al., 2010). Also, xerostomy is another condition that reflects the decrease or the complete absence of saliva (Webb et al., 1998b), reducing the ability of cleaning and buffering of saliva. Furthermore, previous study showed that patients with xerostomy induce changes that reflect in the normal microbial communities, favoring the proliferation of bacteria as *Staphylococcus aureus*, which inhibits the normal adaptation of the commensal fungals (Webb et al., 1998a).

Cigarette smoke may favor CADS, considering the changes that cause in the oral cavity, influencing on saliva, oral commensal bacteria and fungi, especially *Candida*, the main fungal related to CADS (Soysa and Ellepola 2005). Another important factor is the trauma. Although trauma alone does not induce to generalize CADS, it should be considered that trauma acts as a cofactor, favoring the adhesion and penetration of the yeasts in the oral epithelium mucosa of the host (Emami et al., 2008). Denture trauma due to poorly adapted denture is an important cofactor of CADS.

Complete denture wearers are also a risk factor, considering that *Candida* spp. are frequently found on oral mucosa and on denture surfaces (Sánchez-Vargas et al., 2013; Daniluk et al., 2006). In addition, it was observed that the presence of C. albicans in the oral cavity in patients with dentures was higher than in patients who do not use dentures (Daniluk et al., 2006). Furthermore, poor oral hygiene favors the biofilm development (Daniluk et al., 2006), and therefore it is important to have a correct oral hygiene.

A carbohydrate-rich diet also favors the microorganisms adhesion and proliferation, taking into account that the carbohydrates are the primary and preferred nutrient source for *Candida* spp. (Emami et al., 2014), and may modulate biofilm development on denture surface by affecting both structural features and virulence factor in *C. albicans* biofilms (Ene et al., 2012).

Finally, the environmental pH may act as a potential inducer of biofilm development (Santana et al., 2013), and previous study showed that acidic pH (pH 5.5) may be more favorable for biofilm formation (Davis 2003).

Systemic Factors

There are a lot of systemic conditions that may influence the development of CADS. Here, diabetes, chemotherapy, hemophilia, and immunosuppressed patients will be emphasized.

Diabetes mellitus is one of the chronic systemic factors with major influence of the oral environment (Vasconcellos et al. 2014). Considering the lower glycemic control, the high glucose level on oral fluid, and the immune dysregulation, diabetes frequently causes xerostomy, which favors fungal proliferation (Girtan et al., 2009).

Furthermore, patients undergoing chemotherapy are particularly affected by CADS, due to high sensibility of the oral tissues to the toxic effects of chemotherapy. Antineoplastic drugs act on proliferating cells without distinguishing the normal cells from cancerous cells. In this context, the constant cell renewal of the oral mucosa, the complex microbiota (greatly altered with the use of anticancer drugs), xerostomy, neutropenia, and immunosuppression resulted from the treatment facilitated proliferation of *Candida* spp. in the oral environment (Lotfi-Kamran et al., 2009). Hemophilia is another important risk factor for CADS. A previous study showed that 64 % of hemophiliacs' patients had preexisting infections or reduction in salivary flow (Wilberg et al., 2014).

Finally, the major risk factor for the proliferation of *C. albicans* is immunosuppression, which changes the homeostasis of human host. It was revealed that 87.5 % of the HIV-positive patients were *Candida* carriers/positive in saliva (Wilberg et al., 2014).

Clinical Manifestations

There are several forms of oral candidiasis, such as pseudomembranous candidiasis, erythematous candidiasis, angular cheilitis, and chronic hyperplastic candidiasis. Here we will emphasize the CADS, a type of erythematous candidiasis that occurs under a removable denture.

Clinical characteristics may range from no symptoms to severe pain and difficulty swallowing (Lalla et al., 2013; Pereira et al., 2004). The most common signs include changes in color and texture of the mucosa, dry mouth, painful symptomatology, and erythematous aspect (Wilson 1998).

Newton (1962) proposed a classification of the disease based on clinical aspects of the lesions: punctiform hyperemia (class I), diffuse hyperemia (class II), and granular hyperemia (class III) (de Oliveira et al., 2010).

1. Punctiform hyperemia (Class I): hyperemia signs of the minor palatine salivary glands; there is an erythematous punctiform aspect, and small or diffuse areas in palate may be affected.
2. Diffuse hyperemia (Class II): smooth and atrophic mucosa, with erythematous aspect under the denture. It is considered the most common aspect of CADS.
3. Granular hyperemia (Class III): more common in dentures with suction chambers. Affect the central region of the palate, with rough and nodular appearance of the mucosa.

It is important to highlight that the therapeutic test is a widely used diagnostic measure, which consists of prescribing topical antifungals and evaluate if there is a regression of signs and symptoms of the disease, to observe if the clinical manifestations are related to CADS. When there is a regression of the lesion after the treatment, ranging from 7 to 14 days, it may be assumed that the clinical manifestations were associated with CADS (Newton 1962).

Therapy Strategies

The treatment of CADS consists in removing the etiological agent, give instructions to the patient in relation to oral hygiene of denture surface and oral mucosa and treat the affected tissue. In addition, the professional should evaluate the necessity to confect another denture, considering that infected prosthetic devices typically must be removed (Williams and Lewis 2000).

The miconazole 2 % has been successful used, being commercially available in form of gel, and can be applied directly in the denture surface previously cleaned. It should be used 2–3 times a day for 1 or 2 weeks, according to the patient response (Newton 1962). A topical antifungal agent widely used for the treatment of CADS is nistatin, which can be used on the oral mucosa several times a day, being available as a liquid suspension, cream, and pastille (Lalla et al., 2013).

When the therapy via topical antifungal agents does not lead to clinical improvement of the patient, the use of systemic antifungal agents is recommended, especially in immunosuppression patients. The fluconazole (FLZ) has been extensively used, taking into account that it has lower toxicity, it is highly bioavailable in oral formulations, and less expensive in relation to other antifungal agents (Montejo 2011). A single and daily dose is recommended, the first dose being of 400 mg and subsequent daily doses of 100 mg for 1 or 2 weeks (Spellberg et al., 2006). Another systemic antifungal agent is ketoconazole, which is absorbed from the gastrointestinal tract and must be administered in a single dose of 200 mg during 14 days. This is a hepatotoxic drug and can cause cardiac arrhythmias when used in combination with antihistamines or macrolide antibiotics (Ramage et al., 2002). For a long time, amphotericin B was used in the treatment of CADS. However, it is extremely nephrotoxic and is administered intravenously, nowadays being used less in CADS therapy.

Conclusion

The knowledge about *Candida*-associated denture stomatitis is of utmost importance in clinical practice. The professional should recognize the possible risk factors for CADS and the clinical manifestations, in order to indicate the correct treatment for the patients.

References

Cueto A, Martínez R, Niklander S, Deichler J, Barraza A et al (2013) Prevalence of oral mucosal lesions in an elderly population in the city of Valparaiso, Chile. Gerodontology 30(3):201–206

Daniluk T, Tokajuk G, Stokowska W, Fiedoruk K, Sciepuk M et al (2006) Occurrence rate of oral *Candida albicans* in denture wearer patients. Adv Med Sci 51:77–80

Davis D (2003) Adaptation to environmental pH in *Candida albicans* and its relation to pathogenesis. Curr Genet 44(1):1–7

de Oliveira CE, Gasparoto TH, Dionísio TJ, Porto VC, Vieira NA et al (2010) *Candida albicans* and denture stomatitis: evaluation of its presence in the lesion, prosthesis, and blood. Int J Prosthodont 23(2): 158–159

Dorocka-Bobkowska B, Konopka K (2007) Susceptibility of candida isolates from denture-related stomatitis to antifungal agents in vitro. Int J Prosthodont 20(5): 504–506

Emami E, de Grandmont P, Rompré PH, Barbeau J, Pan S et al (2008) Favoring trauma as an etiological factor in denture stomatitis. J Dent Res 87(5):440–444

Emami E, Kabawat M, Rompre PH, Feine JS (2014) Linking evidence to treatment for denture stomatitis: a meta-analysis of randomized controlled trials. J Dent 42(2):99–106

Ene IV, Adya AK, Wehmeier S, Brand AC, MacCallum DM et al (2012) Host carbon sources modulate cell wall architecture, drug resistance and virulence in a fungal pathogen. Cell Microbiol 14(9):1319–1335

Girtan M, Zurac S, Stăniceanu F, Bastian A, Popp C et al (2009) Oral epithelial hyperplasia in diabetes mellitus. Rom J Intern Med 47(2):201–203

Harriott MM, Noverr MC (2011) Importance of *Candida-bacterial* polymicrobial biofilms in disease. Trends Microbiol 19(11):557–563

Jayatilake JA (2011) A review of the ultrastructural features of superficial candidiasis. Mycopathologia 171(4):235–250

Lalla RV, Patton LL, Dongari-Bagtzoglou A (2013) Oral candidiasis: pathogenesis, clinical presentation, diagnosis and treatment strategies. J Calif Dent Assoc 41(4):263–268

Lotfi-Kamran MH, Jafari AA, Falah-Tafti A, Tavakoli E, Falahzadeh MH (2009) *Candida* colonization on the denture of diabetic and non-diabetic patients. Dent Res J (Isfahan) 6(1):23–27

Montejo M (2011) Epidemiology of invasive fungal infection in solid organ transplant. Rev Iberoam Micol 28(3):120–123

Nett JE, Marchillo K, Spiegel CA, Andes DR (2010) Development and validation of an in vivo *Candida albicans* biofilm denture model. Infect Immun 78(9):3650–3659

Newton AV (1962) Denture sore mouth: a possible etiology. Br Dent J 1:357–360

Pereira CM, Pires FR, Corrêa ME, di Hipólito JO, Almeida OP (2004) *Candida* in saliva of Brazilian hemophilic patients. J Appl Oral Sci 12(4):301–306

Ramage G, VandeWalle K, Bachmann SP, Wickes BL, López-Ribot JL (2002) *In vitro* pharmacodynamic properties of three antifungal agents against preformed *Candida albicans* biofilms determined by time-kill studies. Antimicrob Agents Chemother 46(11):3634–3636

Salerno C, Pascale M, Contaldo M, Esposito V, Busciolano M et al (2011) *Candida*-associated denture stomatitis. Med Oral Patol Oral Cir Bucal 16(2):139–143

Sánchez-Vargas LO, Estrada-Barraza D, Pozos-Guillen AJ, Rivas-Caceres R (2013) Biofilm formation by oral clinical isolates of *Candida* species. Arch Oral Biol 58(10):1318–1326

Santana IL, Gonçalves LM, de Vasconcellos AA, da Silva WJ, Cury JA et al (2013) Dietary carbohydrates modulate *Candida albicans* biofilm development on the denture surface. PLoS One 8(5), e64645

Sardi JC, Scorzoni L, Bernardi T, Fusco-Almeida AM, Mendes Giannini MJ (2013) *Candida* species: current epidemiology, pathogenicity, biofilm formation, natural antifungal products and new therapeutic options. J Med Microbiol 62:10–24

Soysa NS, Ellepola AN (2005) The impact of cigarette/tobacco smoking on oral candidosis: an overview. Oral Dis 11(5):268–273

Spellberg BJ, Filler SG, Edwards JE Jr (2006) Current treatment strategies for disseminated candidiasis. Clin Infect Dis 42(2):244–251

Vallejo JA, Sánchez-Pérez A, Martínez JP, Villa TG (2013) Cell aggregations in yeasts and their applications. Appl Microbiol Biotechnol 97(6):2305–2318

Vasconcellos AA, Gonçalves LM, Del Bel Cury AA, da Silva WJ (2014) Environmental pH influences *Candida albicans* biofilms regarding its structure, virulence and susceptibility to fluconazole. Microb Pathog 69–70:39–44

Vazquez JA, Sobel DJ (2002) Mucosal candidiasis. Infect Dis Clin North Am 16(4):793–820

Webb BC, Thomas CJ, Willcox MD, Harty DW, Knox KW (1998a) *Candida*-associated denture stomatitis. Aetiology and management: a review. Part 2. Oral diseases caused by Candida species. Aust Dent J 43(3):160–166

Webb BC, Thomas CJ, Willcox MD, Harty DW, Knox KW (1998b) *Candida*-associated denture stomatitis. Aetiology and management: a review. Part 1. Factors influencing distribution of *Candida* species in the oral cavity. Aust Dent J 43(1):45–50

Wilberg P, Hjermstad MJ, Ottesen S, Herlofson BB (2014) Chemotherapy-associated oral sequelae in patients with cancers outside the head and neck region. J Pain Symptom Manage 48(6):1060–1069

Williams DW, Lewis MA (2000) Isolation and identification of Candida from the oral cavity. Oral Dis 6(1):3–11

Wilson J (1998) The aetiology, diagnosis and management of denture stomatitis. Br Dent J 185(8):380–384

Zissis A, Yannikakis S, Harrison A (2006) Comparison of denture stomatitis prevalence in 2 population groups. Int J Prosthodont 19(6):621–625

Oral Chronic Hyperplastic Candidosis

8

Antonio Adilson Soares de Lima
and Maria Ângela Naval Machado

Abstract

Chronic hyperplastic candidosis/candidiasis (CHC) or Candidal Leukoplakia is a clinical variant of oral candidosis, whose etiology is associated with the fungal pathogen, *Candida albicans*. It is the least common of the three main clinical variants of oral candidosis (pseudomembranous, erythematous, and hyperplastic variants).

The major etiologic agent of the disease is Candida, but other factors may play a contributory role in the pathogenesis of CHC.

Chronic hyperplastic candidosis/candidiasis (CHC) or Candidal Leukoplakia is a clinical variant of oral candidosis, whose etiology is associated with the fungal pathogen, *Candida albicans*. It is the least common of the three main clinical variants of oral candidosis (pseudomembranous, erythematous, and hyperplastic variants).

Oral candidosis lesions were subdivided in primary oral candidosis and secondary oral candidosis. Primary oral candidosis are confined to lesions localized to the oral cavity with no involvement of skin or other mucosa. In secondary oral candidosis, lesions are present in the oral as well as extra-oral sites such as skin (Sitheeque and Samaranayake 2003).

The primary oral candidosis lesions consist of pseudomembranous, erythematous, and hyperplastic variants.

The major etiologic agent of the disease is Candida, but other factors may play a contributory role in the pathogenesis of CHC. Local and systemic factors may act to facilitate the conversion of *C. albicans* in a pathogenic organism.

A local predisposing factor, such as occlusal trauma or friction in commissural leukoplakias, causes a breach of the integrity of the host oral mucosa initiating the CHC (Arendorf et al., 1983). Other factor cited is that smoking habit has a strong correlation with commissural leukoplakia (Beasley 1969). Almost all patients with chronic hyperplastic candidiasis are smokers. More frequently, *Candida albicans* was isolated from the mouths of smokers than from nonsmokers (Arendorf and Walker 1980).

A.A.S. de Lima (✉) • M.Â.N. Machado
Faculty of Dentistry, Federal University of Paraná,
Curitiba, Brazil
e-mail: aas.lima@ufpr.br

E.A.R. Rosa (ed.), *Oral Candidosis: Physiopathology, Decision Making, and Therapeutics*,
DOI 10.1007/978-3-662-47194-4_8

The systemic predisposing factors cited in the pathogenesis of candidosis are diabetes, immunological defects, and nutritional factors.

It is not well established whether the invasion by *Candida* is the primary factor in the development of chronic hyperplastic candidosis, or if the infection by Candida is secondary to localized epithelial alterations (Scully et al., 1994).

CHC has long been associated with the development of oral squamous cell carcinoma, although the role of *Candida* in the process of malignant transformation still remains unclear (Sitheeque and Samaranayake 2003). There are reports of malignancy in 15 % of cases.

Lesions heterogeneous of hyperplastic candidosis, in which the white plaques are intermingled with erythematous areas, have been associated with higher malignant potential (Barrett et al., 1998).

Clinical Characteristics

Clinically, the classic appearance of CHC in the oral mucosa shows a white patch at the commissural regions (Fig. 8.1, 8.2, 8.3, and 8.4), but can also occur at the palate and lateral border of the tongue (Samaranayake et al., 2009). The lesions are symptomless and resistant to scratching varying from small translucent whitish areas (Figs. 8.1 and 8.2) to large opaque plaques (Figs. 8.3 and 8.4) (Reichart et al., 2000).

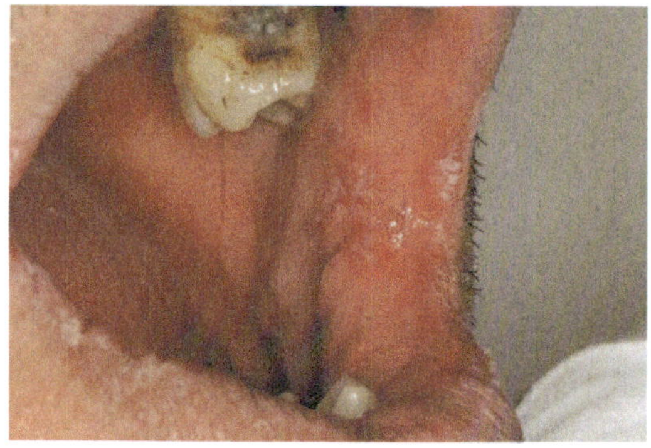

Fig. 8.1 Clinical aspect of chronic hyperplastic candidosis at the commissures and oral mucosa

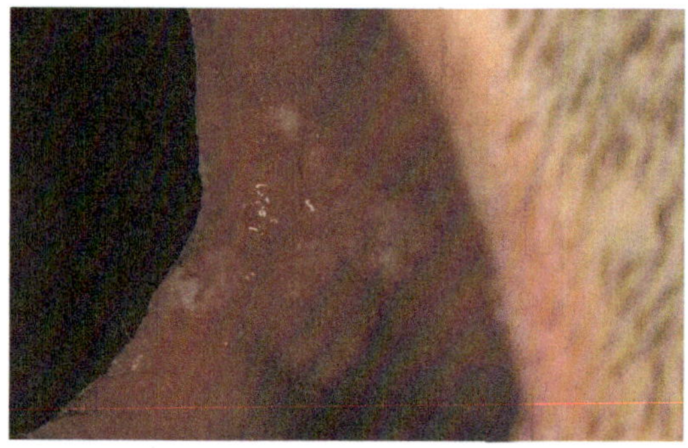

Fig. 8.2 Clinical appearance of plaque-like lesion of right commissural and retrocommissural area

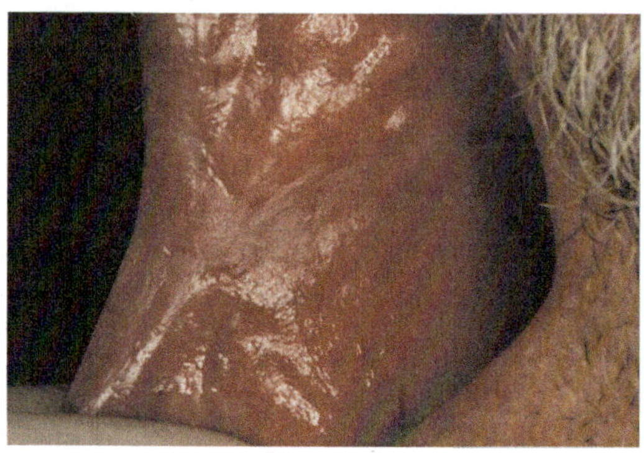

Fig. 8.3 Chronic hyperplastic candidosis at the commissural and retrocommissural area

Diagnosis

In general, the diagnosis of oral candidosis is based on clinical signs and symptoms in conjunction with a complete medical history. Clinical diagnosis is usually confirmed by laboratory tests from clinical samples (Farah et al., 2010). Oropharyngeal swab cultures may demonstrate Candida spp., but, because colonization of the oral mucosa by Candida is common, this is not necessarily diagnostic. Confirmation of a diagnosis of oral candidosis can be accomplished via a 10 % potassium hydroxide slide preparation of a mucosal scraping from a suggestive oral lesion (Thompson et al., 2010). Often, a biopsy is required to establish the diagnosis of oral hyperplastic chronic candidosis and to rule out other white lesions.

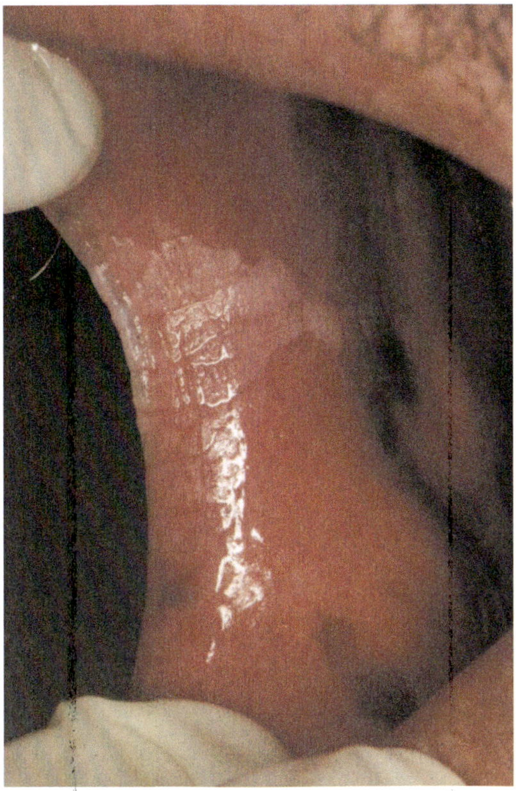

Fig. 8.4 Plaque-like lesion at the commissural and retro-commissural region in oral mucosa

Histopathological Characteristics

The histopathological characteristics of CHC may vary according to their clinical presentation. The candida infection not only causes epithelial hyperplasia, but can also induce epithelial atypias (Shibata et al., 2011).

The following histopathologic features can be found in cases of oral hyperplastic chronic candidosis:

- Hyperplasia of the rete ridges (Fig. 8.5)
- Hyperorthokeratinized or hyperparakeratinized mucosa (Fig. 8.6)
- Chronic inflammatory cells infiltrate (Fig. 8.7)
- Acanthosis (Fig. 8.7)
- Epithelial dysplasia (Fig. 8.7)
- Dyskeratoses (Fig. 8.8)
- Invasion of the hyphae (Fig. 8.9)
- Collections of polymorphonuclear leukocytes (microabscesses)

Histologically, some cases of CHC may mimic squamous cell carcinoma (Saraydaroglu et al., 2010; Tahara, Nibu 2011) and, in particular, verrucous carcinoma. Some authors suggest that those cases that exhibit pronounced epithelial hyperplasia

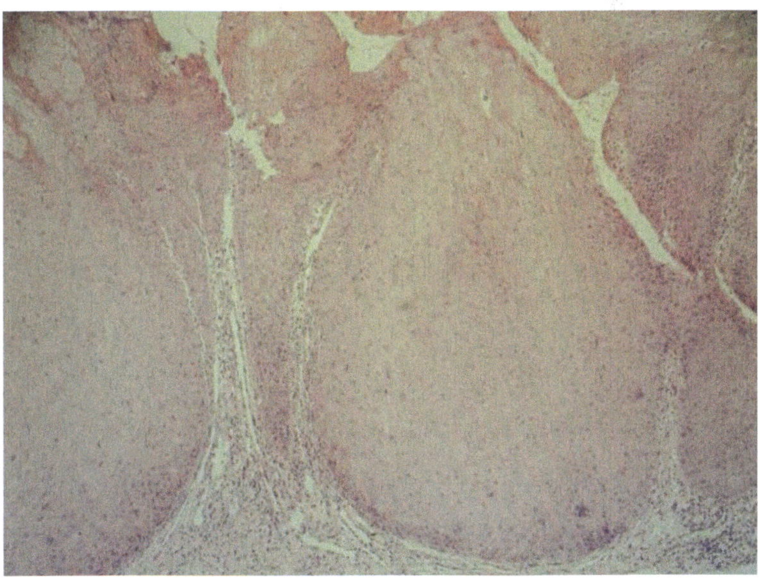

Fig. 8.5 Histopathological aspect of chronic hyperplastic candidosis – epithelial hyperplasia (HE ×10)

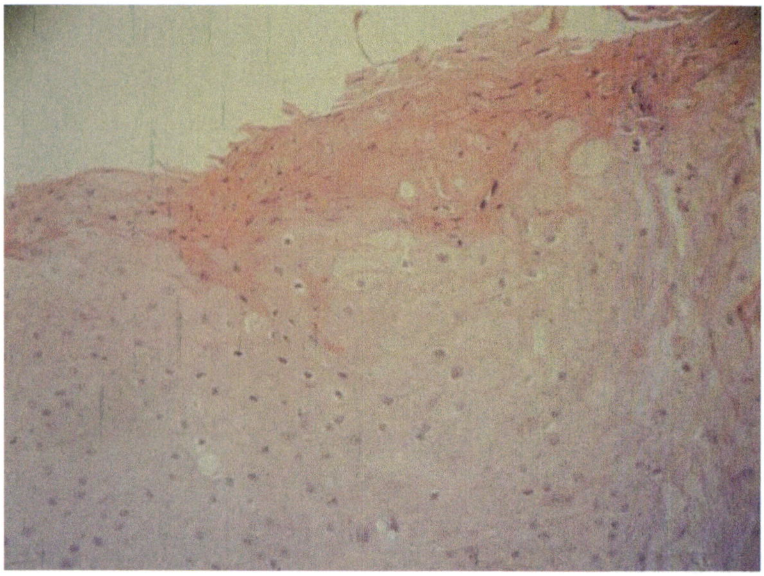

Fig. 8.6 Histopathological aspect of chronic hyperplastic candidosis – hyperparakeratosis (HE ×100)

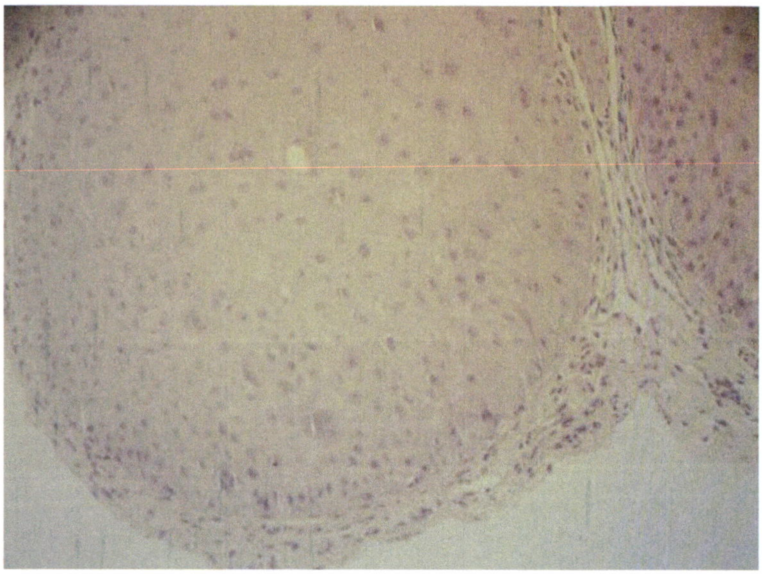

Fig. 8.7 Homogenous chronic hyperplastic candidosis – epithelial dysplasia, acanthosis, hyperchromatism, and chronic inflammatory cell infiltrate in the lamina propria (HE ×100)

and/or verrucous carcinoma-like features should be extensively searched for hyphae or yeasts (Pabuççuoglu et al., 2002) in order to avoid the misdiagnosis of dysplasia or malignancy.

Treatment

The treatment of CHC is practically the same as for other forms of the disease. The recommended treatment initially consists in the elimination of predisposing factors in promoting fungal infection followed by antifungal therapy (Shibata et al., 2011). Cigarette smoking has been considered as the main risk behavior associated with the development of oral chronic hyperplastic candidosis. Thus, elimination of this habit is relevant to successful treatment.

The literature presents different methods of treatment for oral chronic hyperplastic candidosis. The treatment includes medical management in the form of antifungal therapy (Williams et al., 2011) or even topical application of certain agents such as retinoids (Scardina et al., 2009),

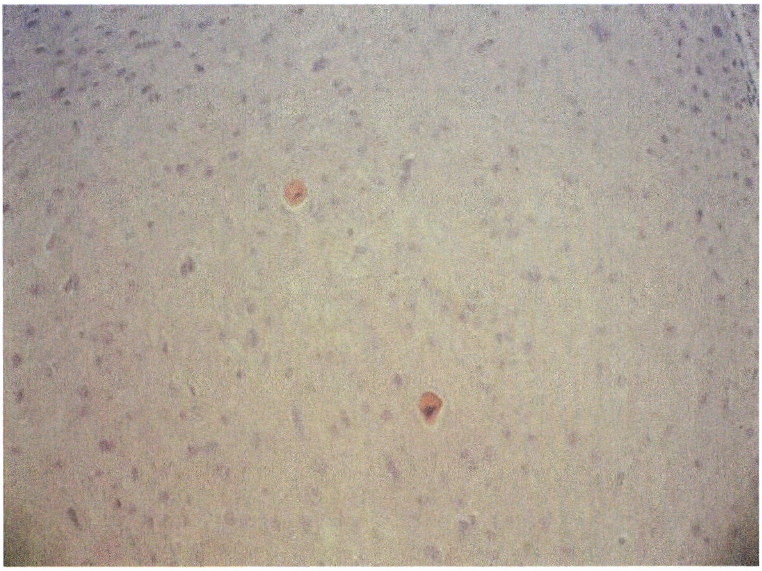
Fig. 8.8 Homogenous chronic hyperplastic candidosis – dyskeratoses (HE ×100)

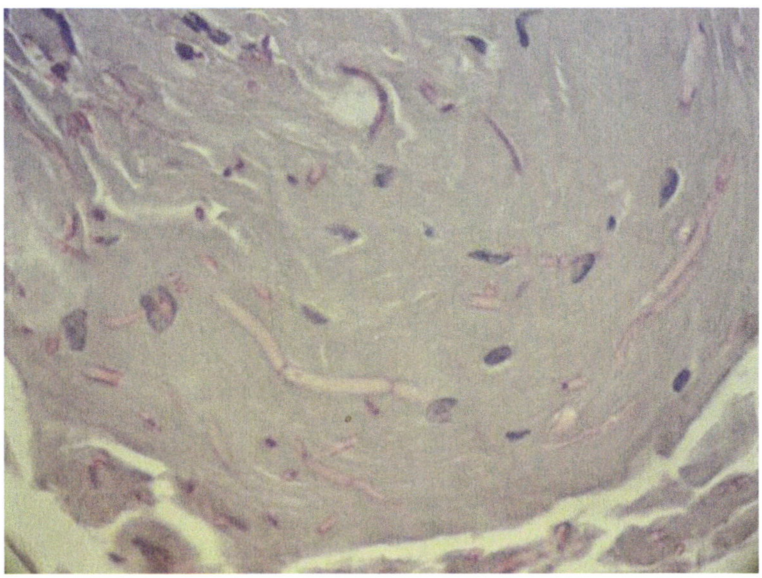
Fig. 8.9 Homogenous chronic hyperplastic candidosis – fungal invasion of the epithelium tissue (PAS ×400)

bleomycin, beta carotene, and surgical methods. Many dentists prefer to begin treatment of lesions using topical and/or systemic before opting for surgical removal.

The treatment of CHC using triazole antifungal drugs (fluconazole) is not always effective to undertake complete remission of lesions and surgical removal of residual lesion may be required. If the lesions are untreated, a minor proportion may demonstrate dysplasia and develop into carcinomas (Holmstrup, Bessermann 1983).

References

Arendorf TM, Walker DM (1980) The prevalence and distribution of Candida albicans in man. Arch Oral Biol 15:1–10

Arendorf TM, Walker DM, Kingdom RJ, Roll JRS, Newcombe RG (1983) Tobacco smoking and denture wearing in oral candidal leukoplakia. Br Dent J 155:340–343

Barrett AW, Kingsmill VJ, Speight PM. The frequency of fungal infection in biopsies of oral mucosal lesions. Oral Dis 1998;4:26–31

Beasley JD III (1969) Smoking and oral moniliasis. J Oral Med 24:83–86

Farah CS, Lynch N, McCullough MJ (2010) Oral fungal infections: an update for the general practitioner. Aust Dent J 55(Suppl 1):48–54
Holmstrup P, Bessermann M (1983) Clinical, therapeutic, and pathogenic aspects of chronic oral multifocal candidiasis. Oral Surg Oral Med Oral Pathol 56(4):388–395
Pabuççuoğlu U, Tuncer C, Sengiz S (2002) Histopathology of candidal hyperplastic lesions of the larynx. Pathol Res Pract 198(10):675–678
Reichart PA, Samaranayake LP, Philipsen HP (2000) Pathology and clinical correlates in oral candidiasis and its variants: a review. Oral Dis 6(2):85–91
Samaranayake LP, Keung Leung W, Jin L (2009) Oral mucosal fungal infections. Periodontology 2000 49:39–59
Saraydaroglu O, Coskun H, Elezoglu B (2010) An interesting entity mimicking malignancy: laryngeal candidiasis. J Int Med Res 38(6):2146–2152
Scardina GA, Ruggieri A, Messina P (2009) Chronic hyperplastic candidosis: a pilot study of the efficacy of 0.18% isotretinoin. J Oral Sci 51(3):407–410
Scully C, El-Kabir M, Samaranayake LP (1994) Candida and oral candidosis: a review. Crit Rev Oral Biol Med 5:125–157
Shibata T, Yamashita D, Hasegawa S, Saito M, Otsuki N, Hashikawa K, Tahara S, Nibu K (2011) Oral candidiasis mimicking tongue cancer. Auris Nasus Larynx 38(3):418–420
Sitheeque MA, Samaranayake LP (2003) Chronic hyperplastic candidosis/candidiasis (candidal leukoplakia). Crit Rev Oral Biol Med 14(4):253–267
Tahara S, Nibu K (2011) Oral candidiasis mimicking tongue cancer. Auris Nasus Larynx 38(3):418–420
Thompson GR 3rd, Patel PK, Kirkpatrick WR, Westbrook SD, Berg D, Erlandsen J, Redding SW, Patterson TF (2010) Oropharyngeal candidiasis in the era of antiretroviral therapy. Oral Surg Oral Med Oral Pathol Oral Radiol Endod 109(4):488–495
Williams DW et al (2011) *Candida* biofilms and oral candidosis: treatment and prevention. Periodontology 2000 55(1):250–265

9 Median Rhomboid Glossitis

Luciana Reis Azevedo Alanis

Abstract

Median rhomboid glossitis (MRG) is defined as the central papillary atrophy of the tongue and it affects 0.25–5.42 % of the population. It consists of a well-defined smooth, reddish, or pinkish area on the dorsum of the tongue located in the midline anterior to the circumvallate papillae. Most of these lesions are asymptomatic, although some patients may complain of persistent pain, irritation, or pruritus. Despite the relative frequency of MRG, little is known about its etiology. There are several predisposing factors associated with MRG such as smoking, denture wearing, diabetes mellitus, as well as candidal infections. If MRG is asymptomatic, no treatment is necessary; if the lesion is painful, a topical antifungal agent may be indicated.

Median rhomboid glossitis (MRG) is defined as the central papillary atrophy of the tongue and it affects 0.25–5.42 % of the population (Bánóczy et al., 1993; Avcu and Kanli 2003). It consists of a well-defined smooth, reddish, or pinkish area on the dorsum of the tongue located in the midline anterior to the circumvallate papillae (Delemarre and van der Waal 1973; McNally and Langlais 1996; Goregen et al., 2011) (Figs. 9.1, 9.2, and 9.3). However, it sometimes appears in the paramedial location (Lago-Méndez et al., 2005). In part, erythema is due to the localized loss of filiform papillae. Most of these lesions are asymptomatic, although some patients may complain of persistent pain, irritation, or pruritus (McNally and Langlais 1996). The surface of the lesion may appear hyperplastic, exophytic, or even sometimes lobulated. MRG may be accompanied by a concomitant contact lesion on the palate (usually the hard palate) (Fig. 9.4), which is called *kissing lesion*. This finding may suggest that these lesions occur as a result of prolonged contact between the Candida-infected midline dorsum of the tongue and the hard palate (Goregen et al., 2011). The diagnosis usually is evident from the clinical appearance of the lesion. MRG generally is regarded as having no malignant potential (McNally and Langlais 1996).

L.R.A. Alanis
Graduate Program in Dentistry, School of Health and Biosciences, Pontifícia Universidade Católica do Paraná, Curitiba, Brazil
e-mail: l.azevedo@pucpr.br

E.A.R. Rosa (ed.), *Oral Candidosis: Physiopathology, Decision Making, and Therapeutics*,
DOI 10.1007/978-3-662-47194-4_9

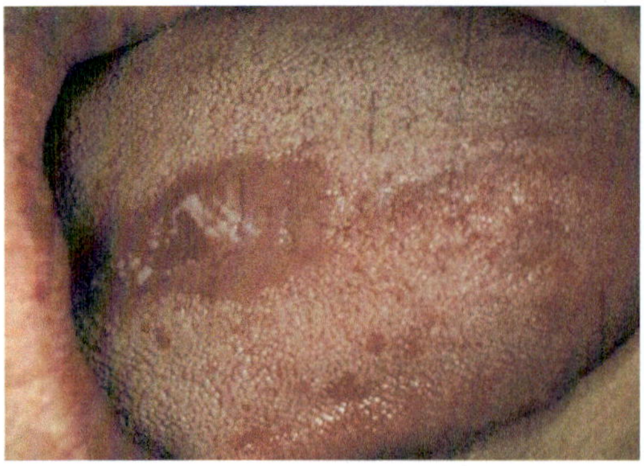

Fig. 9.1 Median rhomboid glossitis. An erythematous, well-defined, elliptical area located posteriorly in the midline of the dorsum of the tongue and anteriorly to the circumvallate papillae

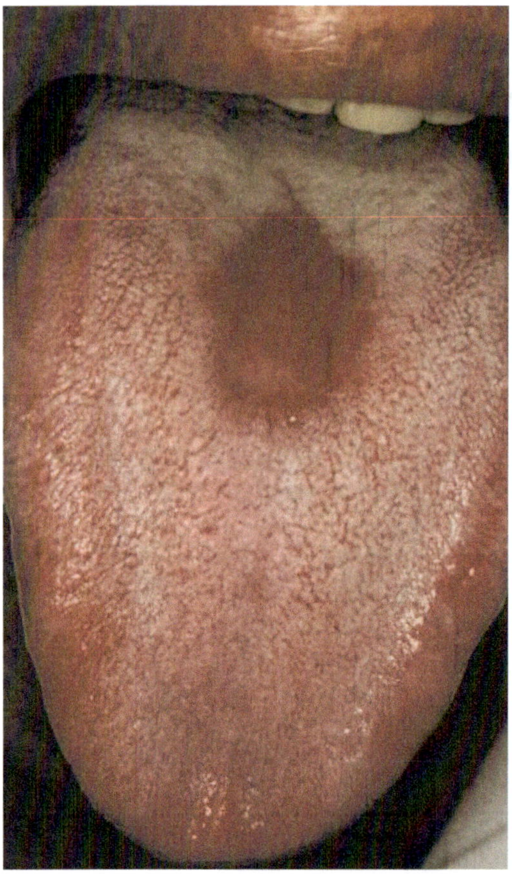

Fig. 9.2 Median rhomboid glossitis. A well-defined smooth, reddish area on the dorsum of the tongue located in the midline anterior to the circumvallate papillae (Courtesy of Prof. Dr. Antonio Adilson Soares de Lima)

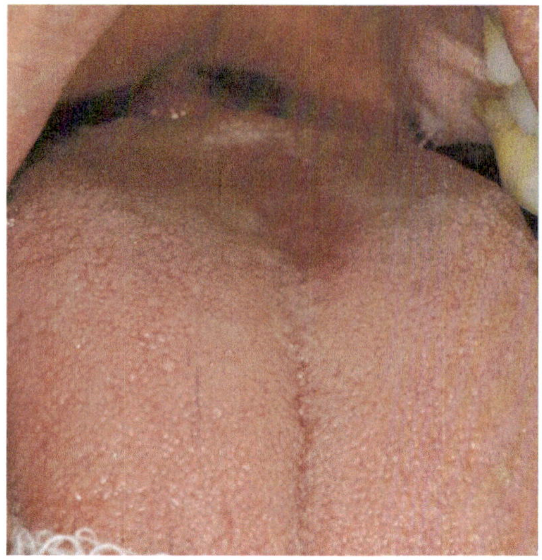

Fig. 9.3 Median rhomboid glossitis. An erythematous, well-defined, elliptical area on the dorsum of the tongue located in the midline anterior to the circumvallate papillae (Courtesy of Prof. Dr. Maria Angela Naval Machado)

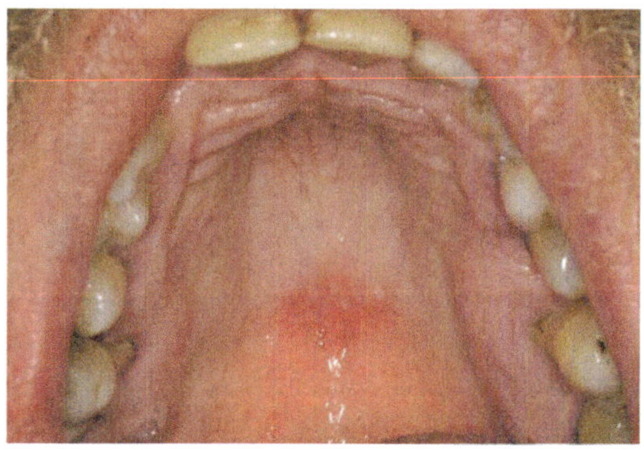

Fig. 9.4 Same patient of Fig. 9.3. Erythematous spot located in the median plane of the hard palate: *kissing lesion* (Courtesy of Prof. Dr. Maria Angela Naval Machado)

Despite the relative frequency of MRG, little is known about its etiology. MRG once was thought to be developmental in origin, although it is seen almost exclusively in adults (Baughman 1971; Cooke 1975). It is now believed to represent an end stage of candidal infection and is similar to papillary hyperplasia of the palate (McNally and Langlais 1996). There are several predisposing factors associated with MRG such as smoking, denture wearing, diabetes mellitus, as well as candidal infections (Espinoza et al., 2003; van der Wal et al., 1986; Soysa and Ellepola 2005). Goregen et al. (2011) observed that although there was a significant association between MRG and Candida and diabetes mellitus, possible risk factors for oral candidosis such as smoking and denture wearing were invalid for MRG. Avcu and Kanli (2003) also observed that the prevalence of MRG was not associated with tobacco use, use of black tea, and oral hygiene index in a Turkish population.

Although there are several studies and hypotheses about the origin of MRG, the importance of Candida to the etiology of this lesion is still controversial because embryological, anatomical, and traumatic factors, and a mixed microbiota may favor the appearance of Candida (Scully et al., 1994; Manfredi et al., 2013). This would explain why the administration of antifungal therapy is sufficient to achieve clinical improvement in some cases and not in another (Samaranayake et al., 2009; Manfredi et al., 2013).

If MRG is asymptomatic, no treatment is necessary; if the lesion is painful, a topical antifungal agent such as nystatin, clotrimazole, or myconazol may be indicated.

Furthermore, application of an aqueous solution of sodium bicarbonate over the lesion can also be conducted (McNally and Langlais 1996).

References

Avcu N, Kanli A (2003) The prevalence of tongue lesions in 5150 Turkish dental outpatients. Oral Dis 9:188–195

Bánóczy J, Rigó O, Albrecht M (1993) Prevalence study of tongue lesions in a Hungarian population. Community Dent Oral Epidemiol 21:224–226

Baughman R (1971) Median rhomboid glossitis: a developmental anomaly? Oral Surg Oral Med Oral Pathol 31(1):56–65

Cooke BE (1975) Median rhomboid glossitis. Candidiasis and not a developmental anomaly. Br J Dermatol 93(4):399–405

Delemarre JFM, van der Waal I (1973) Clinical and histopathologic aspects of median rhomboid glossitis. Int J Oral Surg 2:203–208

Espinoza I, Rojas R, Aranda W, Gamonal J (2003) Prevalence of oral mucosal lesions in elderly people in Santiago, Chile. J Oral Pathol Med 32:571–575

Goregen M, Miloglu O, Buyukkurt MC, Caglayan F, Aktas AE (2011) Median rhomboid glossitis: a clinical and microbiological study. Eur J Dent 5(4):367–372

Lago-Méndez L, Blanco-Carrión A, Diniz-Freitas M, Gándara-Vila P, García-García A, Gándara-Rey JM (2005) Rhomboid glossitis in atypical location: case report and differential diagnosis. Med Oral Patol Oral Cir Bucal 10:123–127

Manfredi M, Polonelli L, Aguirre-Urizar J, Carrozzo M, McCullough M (2013) Urban legends series: oral candidosis. Oral Dis 19(3):245–261

McNally MA, Langlais RP (1996) Conditions peculiar to the tongue. Dermatol Clin 14:257–262

Samaranayake LP, Keung Leung W, Jin L (2009) Oral mucosal fungal infections. Periodontology 2000 49:39–59

Scully C, El-Kabir M, Samaranayake LP (1994) Candida and oral candidosis: a review. Crit Rev Oral Biol Med 5(2):125–157

Soysa NS, Ellepola AN (2005) The impact of cigarette/tobacco smoking on oral candidiasis: an overview. Oral Dis 11:268–273

Van der Wal N, van der Kwast WA, van der Waal I (1986) Median rhomboid glossitis: a follow-up study of 16 patients. J Oral Med 41:117–120

Oral Hairy Leukoplakia

10

Patrícia Carlos Caldeira,
Ana Maria Trindade Grégio,
Mariela Dutra Gontijo de Moura,
and Aline Cristina Batista Rodrigues Johann

Abstract

Oral hairy leukoplakia (OHL) and oral candidiasis (OC) are the most common Human Immunodeficiency Virus (HIV) infection-associated oral diseases, and can act as a marker for immunosuppression. Patients with a prolonged immunodeficiency caused by HIV infection tend to develop OHL and OC, as a progression of Acquired Immune Deficiency Syndrome (AIDS). Few studies describe the joint manifestation of OHL and OC, and its findings are enigmatic. Lower CD4 count and smoking in HIV-infected patients can be independent risk factors for joint manifestation of OHL and OC. OC can be a primary disease or a secondary lesion superimposed on OHL. OHL is a benign oral lesion related to the infection of oral epithelium by Epstein-Barr virus (EBV). It is commonly related with AIDS, but it may also be observed in patients with other immunosuppressed states. OHL is an asymptomatic white plaque on the lateral borders of the tongue and a flat, corrugated, or hairy surface that is not removable when scraped. EBV can be identified through electronic microscopy techniques, in situ hybridization, immunohistochemistry, and polymerase chain reaction; however, the exfoliative cytology can also be used to diagnose OHL. Treatment for OHL is not necessary in most of the patients. Topical treatment such as

P.C. Caldeira, DDS, MSc, PhD • M.D.G. de Moura, DDS, MSc, PhD
Department of Oral Surgery and Oral Pathology, School of Dentistry, Universidade Federal de Minas Gerais, Belo Horizonte, MG, Brazil

A.M.T. Grégio, BPharm, MSc, PhD
A.C.B.R. Johann, DDS, MSc, PhD (✉)
School of Health and Biosciences, Pontifícia Universidade Católica do Paraná, Curitiba, PR, Brazil
e-mail: alinecristinabatista@yahoo.com.br

E.A.R. Rosa (ed.), *Oral Candidosis: Physiopathology, Decision Making, and Therapeutics*,
DOI 10.1007/978-3-662-47194-4_10

retinoid, podophyllin, podophyllin with penciclovir, podophyllin with acyclovir, acyclovir, and gentian violet is most commonly recommended for patients with OHL; but there are other options of treatment such as surgical excision, cryotherapy, and systemic therapy with antiviral drugs.

Oral Candidiasis, Oral Hairy Leukoplakia, and HIV Infection

Oral hairy leukoplakia (OHL) and oral candidiasis (OC) are the most common oral lesions in Human Immunodeficiency Virus (HIV)-infected individuals (Chattopadhyay et al., 2005b), and they can appear as a first manifestation of Acquired Immune Deficiency Syndrome (AIDS) (Reginald and Sivapathasundharam 2010). They have been accepted as markers of immunosuppression (Miziara and Weber 2006; Reginald and Sivapathasundharam 2010; Patton et al., 2013), contributing for the early identification of HIV infection or AIDS (Dias et al., 2012). In addition, OHL and OC can be a sign to warn dentists on the decreasing immunological condition of HIV-infected patients (Moura et al., 2006; Sontakke et al., 2011; Bodhade et al., 2011). Although OC appears to be a superior indicator of immune decline and virologic levels in individuals submit to highly active antiretroviral therapy (HAART), the presence of OHL and OC simultaneously has also been observed as an indicator of low CD4 count and high viral load (Miziara and Weber 2006).

Joint Occurrence of OC and OHL

Although OC and OHL are the two most common oral lesions in HIV-infected patients, few studies describe their joint manifestation (Chattopadhyay and Patton 2007). Eversole et al. (1986) reported 36 cases of OHL in HIV-infected patients with candidiasis detected in 88 % of them. Chattopadhyay and Patton (2007) observed 4.6 % of HIV-infected adults of North Carolina had OHL and OC simultaneously. These authors concluded that lower CD4 count and smoking were independent risk factors for joint manifestation of OC and OHL in HIV-infected individuals. Piperi et al. (2010) found Candida hyphae in 8 of each 10 patients with OHL in HIV-negative patients.

The presence of OHL and OC simultaneously has also been observed as an enigma. OC can be a primary disease or a secondary lesion superimposed on OHL. Because Candida hyphae were not detected all times, the second proposition seems to be sustained (Eversole et al., 1986).

OHL Classification, Etiology, and Risk Indicators

OHL is a benign oral lesion caused by the reactivation of a preceding Epstein-Barr virus (EBV), a herpes virus that frequently shows permanent and asymptomatic latent infection (Cho et al., 2010; Rushing et al., 2011; Dias et al., 2012). In spite of the name "leukoplakia", there are no data to suggest OHL develops into premalignant or malignant lesions, such as oral squamous cell carcinoma (Triantos et al., 1997). It is almost exclusively observed in HIV-infected individuals or with AIDS, but it might also be observed in individuals with other immunosuppressed states, as in patients with leukemia after chemotherapy (Cho et al., 2010), immunosuppressive therapy (Rushing et al., 2011), long-term of anticonvulsant treatment (Gordins et al., 2011), or diabetes mellitus (Milagres et al., 2007).

The assessment of risk indicators for OHL is important to control HIV-infected patients. However, risk indicators described in the literature are variable according to studied population. Risk indicators for OHL in Brazilian HIV-infected adults were viral load, OC, and use of fluconazole or acyclovir, while antiretroviral drugs were shown to be protective for OHL (Moura et al., 2006). CD4 count and antiretroviral drug were relevant risk indicators for OC and

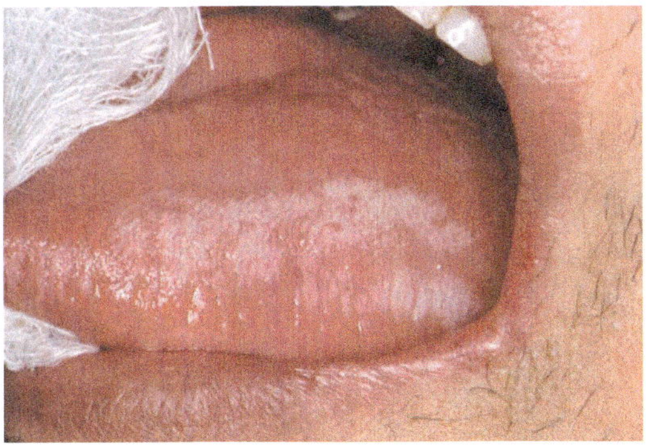

Fig. 10.1 Oral hairy leukoplakia as an asymptomatic white plaque on the lateral borders of the tongue

OHL in HIV-infected adults of North Carolina, but smoking was an important risk indicator just for OC (Chattopadhyay et al., 2005b). In addition, it was verified that low CD4 count and smoking were risk indicators for OC and OHL in HIV-infected adults of North Carolina, while antiretroviral drugs were protective for OC (Chattopadhyay et al. 2005a).

OHL Clinical Characteristics

OHL is characterized by an asymptomatic white plaque on the lateral border of the tongue (Fig. 10.1) (Milagres et al., 2007; Cho et al., 2010; Reginald and Sivapathasundharam 2010; Rushing et al., 2011). It is not removable when scraped and appears as a flat, corrugated, or hairy surface, unilateral or bilateral. OHL rarely involves the floor of the mouth, buccal and labial mucosa, oropharynx, hard and soft palate (Kanitakis et al., 1990; Ficarra et al., 1992; Triantos et al., 1997; Piperi et al., 2010).

OHL Clinical Differential Diagnosis

OHL is most often confused with idiopathic clinical leukoplakia, tobacco-induced leukoplakia, frictional keratosis, edema, lichen planus, galvanic lesions, geographic tongue, maceration, white sponge nevus, oral graft-versus-host disease, and chronic hyperplastic OC (Wescott and Correll 1988; Triantos et al., 1997; Reginald and Sivapathasundharam 2010; Huber 2010). Because of that, it is imperious, the identification of the lesion (Reginald and Sivapathasundharam 2010). Uncharacteristic cases of OHL may be identified by their absence of reaction to antifungal therapy and elimination of other diseases by histologic features (Wescott and Correll 1988).

OHL Histologic Features

OHL clinical identification is indeterminate, so the diagnosis is defined by histologic analysis of tissues from a biopsy sample to verify tissue morphology and identification of replicating EBV (Reginald and Sivapathasundharam 2010).

Histologic features of OHL consist of epithelial hyperplasia with hyperparakeratosis and acanthosis, enlarged and ballooned cells. The cells also show nuclear changes such as: (a) margination of the nuclear chromatin against the nuclear membrane ("nuclear beading"); (b) an eosinophilic central Cowdry type A appearance with a halo homogeneous eosinophilic or basophilic aspect, with marginal chromatin clumping; and (c) nuclei with steel gray or like ground glass aspect, and the chromatin is marginated and clumped (Triantos et al., 1997; Dias et al., 2000; Reginald and Sivapathasundharam 2010).

However, biopsies are invasive procedures and might not be practicable on all patients due to their immune condition. In adding, specific and costly apparatus are necessary to identify EBV, which might not be available (Reginald and Sivapathasundharam 2010). In addition, exfoliative cytology can be used to diagnose and it may be the technique of election for OHL diagnosis for being a simple, reliable, safe, noninvasive, and nontraumatic method (Moura et al., 2007). The keratinocytes with nuclear alterations produced by EBV are present at several layers of the epithelium, including the parakeratin layer, making them readily reachable for sample collection, as an exfoliative analysis (Dias et al., 2012). Overall, the exfoliative cytology allied with EBV in situ hybridization is an easy, useful, and noninvasive diagnostic instrument for OHL (Braz-Silva et al.,

2014). EBV can be identified through electronic microscopy techniques, in situ hybridization, immunohistochemistry, and polymerase chain reaction. An absence of reaction to the antifungal treatment or a verification of an immunosuppressed states may guide the presumptive diagnosis (Moura et al., 2010; Reginald and Sivapathasundharam 2010). In this way, the nuclear alterations produced by EBV and detected by cytopathology is specific and sufficient for the final diagnosis of OHL, independent of the detection of the EBV (Milagres et al., 2007).

OHL Treatment

Treatment for OHL is not necessary in most of the patients (Baccaglini et al., 2007). This lesion frequently resolves in concert with enhanced immunocompetence, as observed in a patient receiving HAART (Huber 2010). The treatments proposed in the literature for OHL include surgical excision, cryotherapy, systemic therapy with antiviral drugs, and topical therapy (Triantos et al., 1997). Topical therapy includes retinoids, podophyllin, podophyllin with penciclovir, podophyllin with acyclovir, acyclovir, and gentian violet (Goh and Lau 1994; Walling et al., 2003; Pastore et al., 2006; Moura et al., 2007; Bhandarkar et al., 2008; Moura et al., 2010). Moura et al. (2010) observed that the treatment with podophyllin with acyclovir cream was more effective in the clinical healing rate for OHL than podophyllin and podophyllin with penciclovir cream, and no recurrent OHL was observed in this first treatment. Additional studies have been conducted on the treatment for OHL with antiviral agents in topical creams (Patton et al., 2013).

References

Baccaglini L, Atkinson JC, Patton LL et al (2007) Management of oral lesions in HIV-positive patients. Oral Surg Oral Med Oral Pathol Oral Radiol Endod 103(suppl 1):S50.e1–S50.e23

Bhandarkar SS, MacKelfresh J, Fried L et al (2008) Targeted therapy of oral hairy leukoplakia with gentian violet. J Am Acad Dermatol 58(4):711–712

Bodhade AS, Ganvir SM, Hazarey VK (2011) Oral manifestations of HIV infection and their correlation with CD4 count. J Oral Sci 53(2):203–211

Braz-Silva PH, Santos RT, Schussel JL et al (2014) Oral hairy leukoplakia diagnosis by Epstein-Barr virus in situ hybridization in liquid-based cytology. Cytopathology 25(1):21–6

Chattopadhyay A, Patton LL (2007) Risk indicators for HIV-associated jointly occurring oral candidiasis and oral hairy leukoplakia. AIDS Patient Care STDS 21(11):825–832

Chattopadhyay A, Caplan DJ, Slade GD et al (2005a) Incidence of oral candidiasis and oral hairy leukoplakia in HIV-infected adults in North Carolina. Oral Surg Oral Med Oral Pathol Oral Radiol Endod 99(1):39–47

Chattopadhyay A, Caplan DJ, Slade GD et al (2005b) Risk indicators for oral candidiasis and oral hairy leukoplakia in HIV-infected adults. Community Dent Oral Epidemiol 33(1):35–44

Cho HH, Kim SH, Seo SH et al (2010) Oral hairy leukoplakia which occurred as a presenting sign of acute myeloid leukemia in a child. Ann Dermatol 22(1):73–76

Dias EP, Rocha ML, Júnior S et al (2000) Oral hairy leukoplakia: histopathologic and cytopathologic features of a subclinical phase. Am J Clin Pathol 114:395–401

Dias EP, Sayed Picciani BL, de Carla Batista Santos V et al (2012) The advantages of oral cytopathology in the early diagnosis of HIV/AIDS: three case reports. Acta Cytol 56(4):453–456

Eversole LR, Jacobsen P, Stone CE et al (1986) Oral condyloma planus (hairy leukoplakia) among homosexual men: a clinicopathologic study of thirty-six cases. Oral Surg Oral Med Oral Pathol 61(3):249–255

Ficarra G, Romagnoli P, Piluso S et al (1992) Hairy leukoplakia with involvement of the buccal mucosa. J Am Acad Dermatol 27(5 Pt 2):855–858

Goh BT, Lau RK (1994) Treatment of AIDS-associated oral hairy leukoplakia with cryotherapy. Int J STD AIDS 5(1):60–62

Gordins P, Sloan P, Spickett GP et al (2011) Oral hairy leukoplakia in a patient on long-term anticonvulsant treatment with lamotrigine. Oral Surg Oral Med Oral Pathol Oral Radiol Endod 111(5):e17–e23

Huber MA (2010) White oral lesions, actinic cheilitis, and leukoplakia: confusions in terminology and definition: facts and controversies. Clin Dermatol 28(3):262–268

Kanitakis J, Zambruno G, Marchand C et al (1990) Oral hairy leukoplakia in AIDS. Histologic and ultrastructural study of 8 cases. Ann Dermatol Venereol 117(5):345–353

Milagres A, Dias EP, Tavares Ddos S et al (2007) Prevalence of oral hairy leukoplakia and epithelial infection by Epstein-Barr virus in pregnant women and diabetes mellitus patients–cytopathologic and molecular study. Mem Inst Oswaldo Cruz 102(2):159–164

Miziara ID, Weber R (2006) Oral candidosis and oral hairy leukoplakia as predictors of HAART failure in Brazilian HIV-infected patients. Oral Dis 12(4): 402–407

Moura MD, Grossmann Sde M, Fonseca LM et al (2006) Risk factors for oral hairy leukoplakia in HIV-infected adults of Brazil. J Oral Pathol Med 35(6):321–326

Moura MD, Guimarães TR, Fonseca LM et al (2007) A random clinical trial study to assess the efficiency of topical applications of podophyllin resin (25%) versus podophyllin resin (25%) together with acyclovir cream (5%) in the treatment of oral hairy leukoplakia. Oral Surg Oral Med Oral Pathol Oral Radiol Endod 103(1):64–71

Moura MD, Haddad JP, Senna MI et al (2010) A new topical treatment protocol for oral hairy leukoplakia. Oral Surg Oral Med Oral Pathol Oral Radiol Endod 110(5):611–617

Pastore L, De Benedittis M, Petruzzi M et al (2006) Efficacy of famciclovir in the treatment of oral hairy leukoplakia. Br J Dermatol 154(2):378–379

Patton LL, Ramirez-Amador V, Anaya-Saavedra G (2013) Urban legends series: oral manifestations of HIV infection. Oral Dis 19(6):533–550

Piperi E, Omlie J, Koutlas IG (2010) Oral hairy leukoplakia in HIV-negative patients: report of 10 cases. Int J Surg Pathol 18(3):177–183

Reginald A, Sivapathasundharam B (2010) Oral hairy leukoplakia: an exfoliative cytology study. Contemp Clin Dent 1(1):10–13

Rushing EC, Hoschar AP, McDonnell JK et al (2011) Iatrogenic oral hairy leukoplakia: report of two cases. J Cutan Pathol 38(3):275–279

Sontakke SA, Umarji HR, Karjodkar F (2011) Comparison of oral manifestations with CD4 count in HIV-infected patients. Indian J Dent Res 22(5):732

Triantos D, Porter SR, Scully C et al (1997) Oral hairy leukoplakia: clinicopathologic features, pathogenesis, diagnosis, and clinical significance. Clin Infect Dis 25(6):1392–1396

Walling DM, Flaitz CM, Nichols CM (2003) Epstein-Barr virus replication in oral hairy leukoplakia: response, persistence, and resistance to treatment with valacyclovir. J Infect Dis 188(6):883–890

Wescott WB, Correll RW (1988) Bilateral white corrugated lesions on the lateral tongue surface. J Am Dent Assoc 116(4):544–546

11 Clinical Correlation of Oral Candidosis and Oral Lichen Planus

João Paulo De Carli, Soluete Oliveira da Silva, Bethânia Molin Giaretta De Carli, Angélica Zanata, Micheline Sandini Trentin, Maria Salete Sandini Linden, and Daniela Cristina Miyagaki

Abstract

Lichen planus is a chronic inflammatory mucocutaneous disease of unclear aetiology. The disease often affects the oral mucosa and may manifest many clinical characteristics, being classified as typical and atypical forms. More importantly, lichen planus has the potential for malignant transformation. Candidosis is the most common disease in the mouth, *Candida albicans* being the main organism found. *Candida* sp. may secondarily infect oral lesions such as leukoplakia, oral lichen planus and squamous cell carcinoma. Patients with oral lichen planus (OLP) frequently present *Candida* infection. Superimposed candidosis lesions can interfere on the diagnosis of OLP, because the organism *Candida albicans* can change the reticular pattern characteristic of OLP. So, the aim of this chapter is to review the literature on the association of candidosis and oral lichen planus.

J.P. De Carli (✉) • S.O. da Silva
Department of Stomatology, University of Passo Fundo, Rio Grande do Sul, Brazil
e-mail: joaoestomatologia@yahoo.com.br

B.M.G. De Carli, MSc
Department of Oral and Maxillofacial Surgery, University of Passo Fundo, Passo Fundo, Rio Grande do Sul, Brazil

A. Zanata
Department of Stomatology, University of Passo Fundo, Passo Fundo, Rio Grande do Sul, Brazil

M.S. Trentin • M.S.S. Linden
Department of Implantology, Post-graduate Program in Dentistry, University of Passo Fundo, Passo Fundo, Rio Grande do Sul, Brazil

D.C. Miyagaki
Department of Endodontics, University of Passo Fundo, Passo Fundo, Rio Grande do Sul, Brazil

Introduction

Candida albicans is one of the most frequently isolated fungi of OLP lesions. Several virulence factors are associated to the pathogenicity of *C. albicans*, including adherence to epithelial or endothelial tissues, phenotypic switching and antigenic modulation as a result of pseudohyphae formation. Previous research also showed that OLP may present some similar clinical manifestations to oral candidiasis (Cai et al. 1997).

Successful colonization of host tissues and infection of microorganisms depend on adherence to the host surfaces. Since the yeast adherence to host surfaces is widely recognized as an essential prerequisite

E.A.R. Rosa (ed.), *Oral Candidosis: Physiopathology, Decision Making, and Therapeutics*, DOI 10.1007/978-3-662-47194-4_11

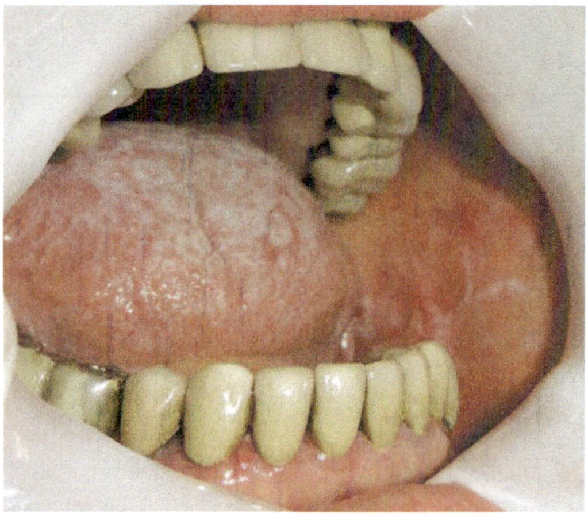

Fig. 11.1 OLP lesions affecting tongue and oral mucosa superimposed by oral candidosis

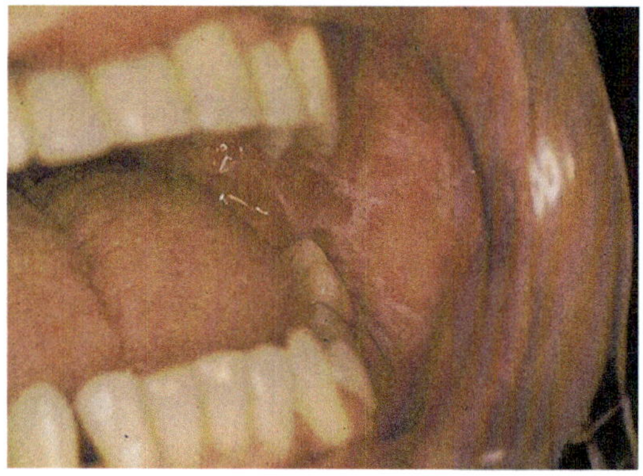

Fig. 11.2 Reticular OLP at the left oral mucosa

in modulating the colonization and infection (Ellepola and Samaranayake 2001a), adhesion plays a crucial role in the permanent attachment of the yeast. A study (Zeng et al. 2009) revealed that the adhesion of *Candida* to erosive OLP is stronger than its adhesion to healthy control tissue. This indicates that *C. albicans* with stronger adhesion influences the permanent attachment, provides qualification for other toxicity factors and participates in the development of the pathological changes (Fig. 11.1).

The objective of this chapter is to review the current literature on the association of candidosis and oral lichen planus, providing important information for a correct diagnosis and adequate treatment of these associated diseases.

Oral Lichen Planus (OLP)

Lichen planus is a relatively common chronic inflammatory disease with a prevalence of oral manifestations between 0.1 and 2.2 % of the population. First described in 1869 by Erasmus Wilson, the disease may involve skin and mucosa, individually or simultaneously. Lesions can be restricted to the mouth or with cutaneous involvement (Navas-Alfaro et al. 2003).

The aetiology of lichen planus has not been completely elucidated; however, it is considered a multifactorial disease mediated by an immunopathological mechanism, particularly involving T lymphocytes (Dorta et al. 2000). In a significant number of cases, the disease is associated with anxiety and depression, according to García-Pola Vallejo et al. (2001). It occurs in patients of both sexes, with a predominance in women, generally over 40 years old (Souza and Rosa 2008).

A total of 50 dermatologists from Bauru/SP/Brazil completed a questionnaire of 19 questions about aetiology, diagnosis and treatment of lichen planus. The main etiological factors reported included idiopathic (22.4 %), psychosomatic (21.5 %), immune (14.0 %) and viral (14.0 %) factors. Other factors related to the disease pathogenesis mentioned by the clinicians were diabetes mellitus, infections, anaemia, genetic predisposition, allergies, smoking habits and sun exposure (Dorta et al. 2000).

According to Souza and Rosa (2008), stress; food such as tomatoes, citrus fruits and spicy dishes; dental procedures; systemic diseases; abuse of alcohol and use of any source of tobacco are associated to periods of exacerbation of the disease. The concern of its association with systemic diseases, especially hepatitis C virus (HCV) infections, is rising in recent years.

The OLP is a disease of polymorphous clinical appearance, being classified as typical or atypical form. The typical form can be divided into reticular (Wickham striae) (Fig. 11.2), popular, plaque and warty. Atypical forms are ulcerated, atrophic, erythematous, erosive (Fig. 11.3) and bullous pigment. In the mouth, it occurs mainly at the buccal mucosa, bilaterally,

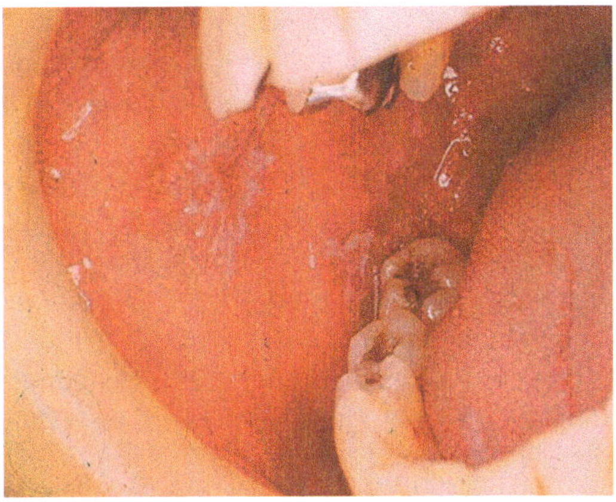

Fig. 11.3 Erosive OLP at the right oral mucosa

at the margin and dorsum of the tongue and at the lip (Souza and Rosa 2008).

Essentially, there are two forms of oral lesions: reticular and erosive. The reticular lichen planus is much more common than the erosive form. However, several studies report the erosive form predominantly, because it is symptomatic and, in many cases, is the only treated variety of OLP. The reticular form usually presents no symptoms and involves the posterior region of the buccal mucosa bilaterally. Other areas of the oral mucosa are likely to be affected, such as the lateral border and dorsum of the tongue, gums, palate and lip vermilion (Navas-Alfaro et al. 2003).

The diagnostic of Lichen planus is performed by biopsy and/or clinical examination of the mouth or skin lesions (Dorta et al. 2000). The lace-like white streaks that appear bilaterally in the posterior region of the buccal mucosa are virtually pathognomonic. Difficulties in diagnostics may arise if the Lichen planus is superimposed by candidosis lesions, because the organism *Candida albicans* can change the reticular pattern characteristic of OLP. Thus, the biopsy of the lesions is often necessary to exclude the hypothesis of other erosive or ulcerative diseases such as systemic lupus erythematosus or chronic ulcerative stomatitis.

Histopathological findings are characteristic of Lichen planus, but may not be specific, since other conditions, such as lichenoid reactions to drugs, may also show similar patterns. Varying degrees of parakeratosis and orthokeratosis may be presented on the surface of the epithelium, depending on the characteristics of the injury (erosive or reticular) from which the sample has been removed. The thickness of the spinous layer can also vary. The interpapillary ridges may be absent or hyperplasic, but are classically pointy shaped or "saw-tooth". The destruction of the basal cell layer of the epithelium (hydropic degeneration) is also evident, accompanied by an intense band-like infiltration, especially T lymphocytes, underlying the epithelium. Degenerate keratinocytes can be seen in the interface area of the epithelium-connective tissue, being called Civatte bodies, colloids or hyaline cytoid (Sugerman et al. 2002). These authors believe that specific and non-specific mechanisms may be involved in the pathogenesis of lichen planus. The former include antigen presentation by keratinocytes of the basal layer and death of antigen-specific cytotoxic T lymphocytes, whereas the latter include mast cell degranulation and activation of matrix metalloproteinases. When these mechanisms are combined, they lead to the accumulation of lymphocytes in the lamina propria underlying the epithelium; disruption of the basement membrane; migration of intraepithelial T lymphocytes; and apoptosis of keratinocytes, which are characteristic of OLP. In addition, the chronic characteristic of the disease can be explained in part by a deficiency in the mechanism of immunosuppression, mediated by transforming beta growth factor.

Regarding the treatment of OLP, 27.6 % of professionals recommend steroids. Some of them reported the use of other therapies for lichen planus reticular with lesions restricted to the oral mucosa, such as cauterization with trichloroacetic acid, rinsing with urea and distilled water, prescription of vitamin A derivatives and tranquilizers (Dorta et al. 2000).

The corticosteroids are the drugs of choice for treatment of lichen planus, because of their ability to modulate the inflammatory and immune response. The topical application and local injection of steroids are being successfully used for controlling the disease. However, the systemic use of corticosteroids is an option for cases presenting severe symptoms. The addition of antifungal drugs improves clinical outcomes. Apparently, this is a consequence of the elimination of secondary growth of *Candida albicans* in tissues affected by OLP. Antifungal drugs also prevent fungal growth associated to the use of corticosteroids (Dorta et al. 2000).

OLP is a local condition presenting defects of epithelial cells. In these cases, the adherence of *Candida* to the oral epithelium is the first step in the infection process and enables the yeast to overcome the normal flushing mechanism of body secretions (De Oliveira et al. 2007; Sherman et al. 2002). *Candida* may act as a secondary pathogen and this super infection can possibly increase the signs and symptoms of OLP, which may be referred as "burning" sensation or discomfort (Kalmar 2007). Dysplastic changes are usually associated to lesions of *Candida* infection mainly because of the potential endogenous nitrosation of this organism (Sumanth et al. 2003).

Oral Candidosis (OC)

Oral candidosis (OC) is the most frequent oral disease (98 % of cases), being an important nosologic entity of the buccal cavity. It is a fungal infection caused by the pathogenic action of *Candida* species, most commonly microorganisms *C. albicans*. These fungi are normally found in the mucous membranes and cause disease only when some growth conditions (predisposing factors) are satisfied. It is estimated that from 30 to 50 % of the population has the microorganism in the mouth and no clinical evidence of infection. The incidence increases with age, reaching close to 60 % of dentate patients over 60 years old (De Oliveira et al. 2007).

According to Stramandinoli (2010), oral candidosis is associated with local and systemic predisposing factors. Local factors comprise poorly sanitized and/or poorly adapted prosthetic restorations or braces; smoking habits; poor oral hygiene and hyposalivation. Systemic predisposing factors include hormonal changes; diseases such as AIDS, diabetes mellitus and other systemic diseases which lead to immunodeficiency; drugs such as corticosteroids, antibiotics and immunosuppressive drugs; and treatments such as head and neck radiotherapy and chemotherapy. Even in the presence of these factors, the invasion of fungus in the superficial layers of the epithelium is mandatory for the disease manifestation.

The candidosis infections are caused by *Candida albicans*. Other members of the genus *Candida*, such as *C. tropicalis*, *C. parapsilosis*, *C. krusei*, *C. guilliermondii*, *C. glabrata*, *C. dubliniensis*, can also be found intra-orally, but only occasionally cause disease. The candidosis may present different clinical aspects, complicating the diagnostic. The infection depends on three factors: the immune status of the host, the environment of the oral mucosa and the resistance of *C. albicans*. The infection can range from mild to fatal when the disease spreads in severely immunocompromised or patients suffering from AIDS (Masaki et al. 2011).

In dental practice, the diagnostic of oral candidosis is usually guided by clinical signs. The definitive identification of the microorganisms is performed by the microbiological diagnosis. For treatment of oral candidosis, various antifungal agents can be used with diverse advantages and disadvantages, as example nystatin, clotrimazole, ketoconazole, fluconazole and itraconazole.

Nystatin, azol-containing therapeutics, e.g. fluconazole, miconazole and ketokonazole, and amphotericin B are the most commonly prescribed drugs for treatment of OC. Alternative substances such as chlorhexidine have both antibacterial and antimycotic effects (Ellepola and Samaranayake 2001b) and colostrum-containing products may have an antimycotic effect as well (Pedersen et al. 2002). *C. krusei* is natively resistant to azol-containing products and *C. glabrata* and *C. dubliniensis* have a weak response to this therapeutics. Thus, selection of resistant *Candida* species after medical treatment can occur (Isham and Ghannoum 2010). The production of nitrosamine by *C. albicans* is pointed out as a possible reason for the higher potential for malignization presented by the non-homogeneous leukoplakias in comparison to the homogeneous leukoplakias (Krogh et al. 1987a). In addition to the morbidity, this is the reason for antimycotic treatment in secondary *Candida* infections in OLP lesions.

Candida is commonly found in oral mucosal lesions and generally causes no problem in healthy people. Overgrowth of *Candida*, however, can lead to local discomfort, an altered taste sensation, dysphagia from oesophageal overgrowth, resulting in poor nutrition, slow recovery and prolonged hospital stays (Akpan and Morgan 2002).

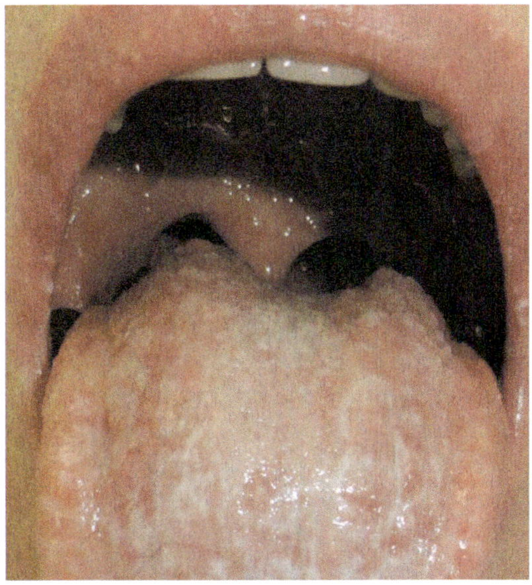

Fig. 11.4 Reticular OLP associated to pseudomembranous candidosis in the tongue

Association of OLP to OC

Oral candidosis (OC) is subdivided into primary and secondary. Secondary infections are superimposed on other diseases of the oral mucous membranes, such as oral lichen planus (OLP), a chronic inflammatory disease. The histopathological characteristics of OLP include hyperkeratinization (Pindborg et al. 1997), which may contribute to a predisposition for *Candida* infection. Erythematous or pseudomembranous areas in OLP can be a manifestation of the disease itself or a result of superimposed candidosis. Both cases are associated to morbidity, suffering and pain (Figs. 11.4 and 11.5) (Scully et al. 1998; Williams et al. 2011).

Candida has been found in 37.0–76.7 % of OLP cases (Krogh et al. 1987b; Jainkittivong et al. 2007). The treatment of OLP with steroids is known to lead to secondary yeast infection, which may complicate the treatment. *C. albicans*, *C. glabrata* and *C. tropicalis* were isolated from OLP lesions treated with topical steroids. Studies have shown that OLP patients suffer from OC and that *C. albicans* is the microorganism most frequently found in OLP patients (Jainkittivong et al. 2007).

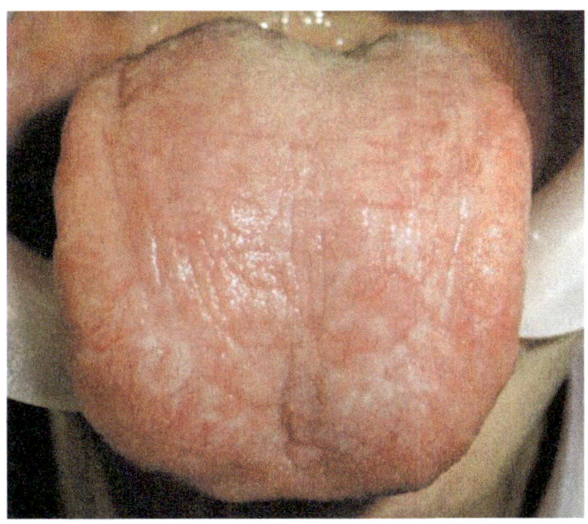

Fig. 11.5 Case of Fig. 11.4 after treatment with nystatin (100,000 IU) three mouthwashes per day during 2 weeks. Note a significant clinical improvement

Kragelund et al. (2013) performed a study to identify correctly the species of *Candida* present in patients with OLP in order to adequate the antifungal treatment, since different *Candida* species have diverse susceptibility to antifungal drugs. Therefore, conventional cytosmear and culture tests were compared to genetic diagnostic. According to the authors, *Candida* species found in oral rinse and agar culture test were different from the samples collected by exfoliative cytology of the mucosa lesion using cytobrush. The exfoliative cytology of the mucosa lesion was able to detect more non-albicans species. Unexpectedly, *Candida dubliniensis* was found to be overrepresented in patients with a history of antimycotic treatment, which indicates iatrogen unintentional selection. An alternative therapy could be suggested for 27 % of the 22 OLP patients receiving treatment, using an improved technique of diagnostic. Correct fungal identification is critical to initiate adequate antimycotic therapy, avoiding the selection of non-albicans species.

In another study, which examined the prevalence of *Candida* species in erosive lesions of OLP, *Candida* species was observed in both healthy participants and in patients with OLP. There was no significant difference between these two groups. Since no significant differences were found between the groups, *Candida* has not been confirmed as an etiologic factor of erosive lichen planus (Mehdipour et al. 2010).

Candida infection has been observed in 17.4 % of ulcerated and 16.4 % of non-ulcerated OLP cases (Hatchuel et al. 1990). Some special genotypic profiles and virulence attributes of *C. albicans* might have a contribution to the development and progression of OLP (Mehdipour et al. 2010; Zeng et al. 2004).

Masaki et al. (2011) detected and identified *Candida* species in samples from the oral mucosa, dorsal surface of the tongue and supragingival plaque of patients with OLP. The authors concluded that healthy individuals with OLP are more prone to have oral colonization of *Candida*, and C. non-albicans species are specifically present in patients with this condition.

Presence of *Candida* spp. was confirmed in 0–17 % of biopsies of OLP, without considering the type of clinical manifestation (erosive or non-erosive lesions) (Hatchuel et al. 1990). A recent study (Zeng et al. 2009) showed higher prevalence of *Candida* spp. in patients presenting the erosive form of OLP (72 %) than the non-erosive form (28 %).

The study of Holmstrup and Dabblesteen (1974) investigated the prevalence and distribution of *Candida* spp. in biopsies of OLP presenting hiperortoqueratose and hyperparakeratosis. The research concluded that OLP lesions lower susceptibility to infection by *Candida* species than other studies since *Candida* was found in only 1 of 43 cases.

Lipperheide et al. (1996) performed a research on the prevalence of colonization by *Candida* species in patients presenting oral leukoplakia, LPB or without oral lesions. The authors observed that the prevalence of yeasts colonization was higher for patients with oral leukoplakia (54.3 %; 19 of 35) and for the group of individuals without oral lesions (45.3 %; 43 of 95) than for the OLP patients (35.3 %; 12 of 34).

Vuckovic et al. (2004) investigated the presence of *Candida* spp. in lesions with malignant potential, especially oral leukoplakia and OLP. *Candida* spp. was found in 3 (25 %) of a total of 12 lesions of oral leukoplakia, and 4 (44 %) of 9 cases of OLP. The presence of yeasts was confirmed in 82 % of patients with oral leukoplakia and 37 % of patients with OLP. The dominant species were *Candida albicans* in both lesions, but *C. tropicalis*, *C. pintolopesii*, *Torulopsisglabrata*, and *Saccharomyces ceresivae* were also found.

Lipperheide et al. (1996) studied the prevalence of *Candida* colonization in patients with OLP, oral leukoplakia and individuals without oral lesions. The authors examined a total of 116 patients (25 with oral leukoplakia, 17 with OLP and 74 individuals without oral lesions). *C. albicans* was the predominant species found in all groups, confirming 76 % cases in patients presenting oral leukoplakia, 88.2 % in individuals with OLP and 60.8 % in individuals without oral lesions. Other species, such as *C. famata*, *C. tropicalis*, *C. parapsilosis*, *C. guilliermondii*, *Rhodotorularubra*, and *Trichosporoncapitatun,* were identified in lesions of oral leukoplakia and OLP. *C. glabrata*, *Cryptococcusalbidus*, *C. krusei*, *C. lipolytica*, *C. intermediate* and *C. rugosa* were also observed in individuals without oral lesions.

In a study assessing the prevalence of *Candida* infection in OLP lesions, 15 patients (44.11 %) of a total of 34 presented *Candida*-positive culture on Sabouraud's dextrose agar medium. None of the 34 histological sections of OLP showed *Candida* hyphae using acid-Schiff staining. No significant association of *Candida* and lichen planus symptoms and patterns were found. The authors concluded that *Candida* infection in OLP patients was not significant (Shivanandappa et al. 2012).

Another study (Spolidorio et al. 2003) determined the prevalence of *Candida* sp. infection in 832 biopsies of oral mucosal lesions, analysing the presence of *Candida* sp. in malignant lesions and lesions with various degrees of dysplasia. Results showed a positive association of *Candida* infection to epithelial dysplasia; mild, moderate and severe squamous cell carcinoma; and hyperkeratosis. Inflammatory fibrous hyperplasia, lichen planus and pyogenic granuloma were not associated to fungal infections. The authors concluded that there was a positive correlation between yeast infection and dysplastic lesions and carcinoma, occurring more frequently in males. These data do not indicate whether the fungus causes epithelial dysplasia and carcinoma, but confirmed the presence of *Candida* in these lesions.

Researches performed in the 1960s were the first reports of a possible association between *Candida* spp. and oral cancerization. In the 1970s, some studies have found strong evidence of the link of *Candida albicans* (specifically) to the oral cancer development (McCullough et al. 2002). For Nagy et al. (1998), the frequency of *Candida* spp., mainly *Candida albicans,* is higher at the areas affected by oral carcinomas than in healthy tissues. In addition to the fact that the OLP is a lesion with carcinogenic potential, such finding suggests that infection by *Candida* fungus is more frequent in OLP lesions than in patients without these lesions.

The study of Barrett et al. (1998) found significant association of fungal infection to the presence of oral lesions with histologically confirmed epithelial dysplasia. This study suggests an interaction between oral infection by yeast, especially *Candida* species, and the development of oral epithelial dysplasia and neoplasia.

The yeast infection's mechanism of action is responsible for the development and progression of dysplasia; however, it remains unclear (McCullough et al. 2002). A study in animals found that *Candida* species have a potential ability for endogenous production of nitrosamines, which are carcinogenic in the oral mucosa (Reibel 2003).

The endogenous nitrosamines metabolism by *Candida* species is observed primarily by *Candida albicans*. These nitrosamines may be associated directly or indirectly to the activation of specific oncogenes, which are responsible for malignant transformation (Sitheeque and Samaranayake 2003; Dwivedi et al. 2009).

Some authors suggest the use of antifungal agents in some cases of OLP to reduce the potential production of carcinogenic N-nitrosobenzylmethylamine by *C. albicans* (Krogh et al. 1987b). It is difficult to establish whether a synergistic premalignant effect would occur in cases of exposure to potentially carcinogenic substances (contributing external risk factors) and persistence of OLP (intrinsic risk factor) (Mehdipour et al. 2010).

Although there are many studies demonstrating the association of *Candida* spp. to oral carcinogenesis (including precancerous lesions, such as OLP), this link is still questionable, needing further study (Meurman and Uittamo 2008).

Final Considerations

Based on the literature reviewed, a higher prevalence of *Candida* yeast infection in patients with OLP when compared to individuals without the disease was suggested. However, whether this infection is a cause or a consequence of OLP lesions remains still unclear, needing further longitudinal clinical and laboratory studies.

References

Akpan A, Morgan R (2002) Oral candidosis. Postgrad Med J 78:455–459

Barrett AW, Kingsmill VJ, Speight PM (1998) The frequency of fungal infection in biopsies of oral mucosal lesions. Oral Dis 4(1):2631

Cai HX, Tong LW, Zhu GY (1997) Triamcinoloneacetonide and antifungal in treatment of oral lichen planus. J Den Pre Treat 5:14–16

De Oliveira MAM, Carvalho LP, Gomes MS, Bacellar O, Barros TF, Carvalho EM (2007) Microbiological and immunological features of oral candidosis. Microbiol Immunol 51(8):713–719

Dorta RG, Colaço CS, Costa CG, Oliveira DT (2000) Conduta médica em pacientes com líquen plano cutâneo e bucal. Rev FacOdontol Bauru 8(3/4):23–28

Dwivedi PP, Mallya S, Dongari-Bagtzoglou A (2009) A novel immunocompetent murine model for *Candida*

albicans promoted oral epithelial dysplasia. Med Mycol 47(2):157–167
Ellepola ANB, Samaranayake LP (2001a) Investigative methods for studying the adhesion and cell surface hydrophobicity of Candida species: an overview. Microbial Ecol Health Dis 13:46–54
Ellepola AN, Samaranayake LP (2001b) Adjunctive use of chlorhexidinein oral candidoses: a review. Oral Dis 7(1):11–17
García-Pola Vallejo MJ, Huerta G, Cerero R, Seoane JM (2001) Anxiety and depression as risk factors for oral lichen planus. Dermatology 203(4):303–307
Hatchuel DA, Peters E, Lemmer J, Hille JJ, McGraw WT (1990) Candidal infection in oral lichen planus. Oral Surg Oral Med Oral Pathol 70(2):48–54
Holmstrup P, Dabblesteen E (1974) The frequency of Candida in oral lichen planus. Scand J Dent Res 82(8):584–587
Isham N, Ghannoum MA (2010) Antifungal activity of miconazole against recent Candida strains. Mycoses 53(5):434–437
Jainkittivong A, Kuvatanasuchati J, Pipattanagovit P, Sinheng W (2007) Candida in oral lichen planus patients undergoing topical steroid therapy. Oral Surg Oral Med Oral Pathol Oral Radiol Endod 104:61–66
Kalmar JR (2007) Diagnosis and management of oral lichen planus. J Calif Dent Assoc 35(6):405–411
Kragelund C, Kieffer-Kristensen L, Reibel J, Bennett EP (2013) Oral candidosis in lichen planus: the diagnostic approach is of major therapeutic importance. Clin Oral Invest 17:957–965
Krogh P, Holmstrup P, Thorn JJ, Vedtofte P, Pindborg JJ (1987a) Yeast species and biotypes associated with oral leukoplakia and lichen planus. Oral Surg Oral Med Oral Pathol 63:48–54
Krogh P, Hald B, Holmstrup P (1987b) Possible mycological etiology of oral mucosal cancer: catalytic potential of infecting Candida albicans and other yeasts in production of N-nitrosobenzylmethylamine. Carcinogenesis 8:1543–1548
Lipperheide V, Quindós G, Jimenéz Y, Pontón J, Bagán-Sebastián JV, Aguirre JM (1996) Candida biotypes in patients with oral leukoplakia and lichen planus. Mycopathologia 134(2):75–82
Masaki M, Sato T, Sugawara Y, Sasano T, Takahashi N (2011) Detection and identification of non-*Candida albicans* species in human oral lichen planus. Microbiol Immunol 55:66–70
McCullough M, Jabera M, Barrett AW, Baina L, Speight PM, Porter SR (2002) Oral yeast carriage correlates with presence of oral epithelial dysplasia. Oral Oncol 38(4):391–393
Mehdipour M, Zenouz AT, Hekmatfar S, Adibpour M, Bahramian A, Khorshidi R (2010) Prevalence of Candida species in OLP. JODDD 4(1):14–16
Meurman JH, Uittamo J (2008) Oral micro-organisms in the etiology of cancer. Acta Odont Scand 66(6):321–326
Nagy KN, Sonkodi I, Szoke I, Nagy E, Newman HN (1998) The microflora associated with human oral carcinomas. Oral Oncol 34(4):304–308
Navas-Alfaro SE, Fonseca EC, Guzmán-Silva MA, Rochael MC (2003) Análise comparativa entre líquen plano oral e cutâneo. J Bras Patol Med Laboratorial 39(4):351–360
Pedersen AM, Andersen TL, Reibel J, Holmstrup P, Nauntofte B (2002) Oral findings in patients with primary Sjogren's syndrome and oral lichen planus – a preliminary study on the effects of bovine colostrum-containing oral hygiene products. Clin Oral Investig 6(1):11–20
Pindborg JJ, Reichart PA, Smith CJ, Van Der Waal I (1997) Histological typing of cancer and precancer of the oral mucosa. WHO, Springer, Berlin
Reibel J (2003) Prognosis of oral pre-malignant lesions: significance of clinical, histopathological, and molecular biological characteristics. Crit Rev Oral Biol Med 14(1):47–62
Scully C, Beyli M, Ferreiro MC et al (1998) Update on oral lichen planus: etiopathogenesis and management. Crit Rev Oral Biol Med 9(1):86–122
Sherman RG, Prusinski L, Ravenel MC, Joralmon RA (2002) Oral candidosis. Quintessence Int 33:521–532
Shivanandappa SG, Ali IM, Sabarigirinathan C, Mushannavar LS (2012) *Candida* in oral lichen planus. JIAOMR 24(3):182–185
Sitheeque MAM, Samaranayake LP (2003) Chronic hyperplastic candidosis/candidosis (candidal leukoplakia). Crit Rev Oral Biol Med 14(4):253–267
Souza FAC, Rosa LEB (2008) Líquen Plano Bucal: considerações clínicas e histopatológicas. Rev Bras Otorrinolaringol 74(2):284–292
Spolidorio LC, Martins VRG, Nogueira RD (2003) Spolidorio DMP. Freqüência de Candidasp em biópsias de lesões da mucosa bucal Pesqui. Odontol Bras 17(1):89–93
Stramandinoli RT (2010) Prevalência de candidose bucal em pacientes hospitalizados e avaliação dos fatores de risco. Rev Sul-Bras Odontol 7(1):66–72
Sugerman PB, Savage NW, Walsh LJ, Zhao ZZ, Zhou XJ, Khan A et al (2002) The pathogenesis of oral lichen planus. Crit Rev Oral Biol Méd 13(4): 350–365
Sumanth KN, BalajiRao B, Mamatha GP, Mujeeb A (2003) Presence of candida in oral lichen planus and leukoplakia. JIAOMR 15(4):154–157
Vuckovic N, Bokor-Bratic M, Vuckovic D, Picuric I (2004) Presence of Candida albicans in potentially malignant oral mucosal lesions. Arch Oncol 12(1):51–54
Williams DW, Kuriyama T, Silva S, Malic S, Lewis MA (2011) Candida biofilms and oral candidosis: treatment and prevention. Periodontology 55(1):250–265
Zeng X, Chen QM, Nie MH, Li BQ (2004) The attribute of Candida albicans isolates from patients with oral lichen planus. Zhonghua Kou Qiang Yi XueZaZhi 39:149–152
Zeng X, Hou X, Wang Z, Jiang L, Xiong C, Zhou M et al (2009) Carriage rate and virulence attributes of oral Candida albicans isolates with oral lichen planus: a study in a ethnic Chinese cohort. Mycoses 52(2): 161–165

Association of *Candida* with Linear Gingival Erythema in HIV-Infected Subjects

12

Chaminda Jayampath Seneviratne
and Ruwan Duminda Jayasinghe

Abstract

Linear gingival erythema (LGE) in HIV patients has a contentious association with *Candida* infection. Although now it is widely accepted that *Candida* contributes to the occurrence of LGE, still some controversy exists in the nature of its association as an aetiological agent. We will briefly discuss the clinical picture of LGE. This will be followed by an update on insight of microbial association with the lesion, prevalence of LGE, diagnosis and treatment. The current hypothesis and proposed mechanism of the LGE are then discussed.

HIV-Associated Oral Candidiasis and Linear Gingival Erythema

From its origin in the early 1980s, human immunodeficiency virus (HIV) has infected millions of humans causing more than 30 million deaths worldwide due to the development of acquired immunodeficiency syndrome (AIDS) (Ryder et al. 2012). It seems that peak of HIV/AIDS pandemic has already passed and now the disease has largely stabilized due to the introduction of highly active anti-retroviral therapy (HAART) in 1996. However, still more than 34 million of people are living with HIV infection. Hence, HIV infection and AIDS continue to have catastrophic global medical and social effects, especially in the regions where prevalence is relatively high, such as in sub-Saharan Africa, Central and South-East Asia, Eastern Europe and South America. HAART has significantly reduced the mortality of HIV/AIDS patients. The mortality index has fallen from 97.4 in 1984 to 19.8 % in 2001. On the other hand, it means there is a considerable number of HIV-infected immune-compromised people live in the world who are susceptible to opportunistic infections at any time of their life. Therefore, it is important to keep abreast of the HIV/AIDS-associated infectious diseases.

The oral manifestations of HIV infection are associated with reduced CD4+ T-lymphocyte levels. In addition, factors such as plasma HIV RNA levels greater than 3,000 copies/mL, xerostomia, poor oral hygiene and smoking have also

C.J. Seneviratne (✉)
Oral Sciences, Faculty of Dentistry, National University of Singapore, Singapore
e-mail: jaya@nus.edu.sg

R.D. Jayasinghe
Department of Oral Medicine and Periodontology, Faculty of Dental Sciences, University of Peradeniya, Peradeniya, Sri Lanka

E.A.R. Rosa (ed.), *Oral Candidosis: Physiopathology, Decision Making, and Therapeutics*,
DOI 10.1007/978-3-662-47194-4_12

been suggested as the predisposing factors for the HIV-related oral manifestations (Nittayananta et al. 2001; Reznik 2005). HIV-infected patients are prone to various forms of oral opportunistic infections that are not usually seen among immune-competent patients. Therefore, oral manifestations are considered as a predictor of full-blown AIDS status of the HIV patients (Reznik 2005). Oral candidiasis was considered a hallmark of AIDS-defining lesions in the early days of HIV/AIDS epidemics (Axéll et al. 1993; Reichart 2003). Oral candidiasis occurs in several guises in HIV/AIDS patients such as pseudomembraneous, erythematous, atrophic, hyperplastic and angular chelitis (Ceballos-Salobrena et al. 2004). In general, 50–90 % of all HIV-positive persons suffer from oral candidiasis at some point, particularly when progressing towards full-blown AIDS (Samaranayake et al. 2009). Higher prevalence of oral candidiasis in HIV patients is due to the multiplicity of aforementioned predisposing factors that facilitate the conversion of commensal *Candida* to a parasitic status (Samaranayake et al. 2009). Therefore, development of oral candidiasis as an oral manifestation of HIV-infected patients is considered a predictor of the patient's progression into full-blown ADIS status. Hence, almost all HIV-infected patients in AIDS status had at least one variant of oral candidiasis prior to the introduction of HAART. Exact percentage of oral candidiasis in HIV patients is difficult to determine due to variations in the study designs. Generally, HAART has considerably reduced the incidence of oral candidiasis in HIV patients (Coogan et al. 2005; Cerqueira et al. 2010; Goncalves et al. 2013). On the other hand, some studies report a significant reduction in hyperplastic and pseudomembranous variants of the disease with a compensatory increase in erythematous candidiasis (Ceballos-Salobrena et al. 2004).

Linear gingival erythema (LGE) in HIV patients has a contentious association with *Candida* infection. Although now it is widely accepted that *Candida* contributes to the occurrence of LGE, still some controversy exists in the nature of its association as an aetiological agent. We briefly discuss the clinical picture of LGE. This will be followed by an update on insight of microbial association with the lesion, prevalence of LGE, diagnosis and treatment. The current hypothesis and proposed mechanism of the LGE are then discussed.

LGE was first reported by Winkler and Murray in 1987 as one of the oral manifestation of HIV/AIDS patients (Winkler and Murray 1987). As the names denotes, LGE appears as a distinct erythematous band along the gingival margin and known as "red band gingivitis" in layman's term (Axéll et al. 1993) (Fig. 12.1). Later studies defined the lesion as marginal erythema because the lesion appears as a band of significant erythema at least 2 mm in thickness, distinctly demarcated from the adjacent gingiva and continuous from papilla to papilla (Lamster et al. 1994). However, LGE may also present as diffuse or petechial patches and the size may vary from 1 or 2 mm to several millimetres of diffused lesion in the attached gingiva and free gingiva (Reznik 2005). It is usually seen in the anterior teeth, but may extend to other parts of the gingiva as a generalized lesion (Reznik 2005). Bleeding and pain are not common clinical features, although some studies have described those occasionally.

LGE was first reported as HIV-associated gingivitis. On the contrary, the term HIV-associated periodontitis was given to a more destructive type of gingival manifestation associated with HIV infection. HIV-associated periodontitis progresses rapidly with ulceration, necrotic gingiva and is often painful. In subsequent classifications, it was renamed as necrotizing ulcerative

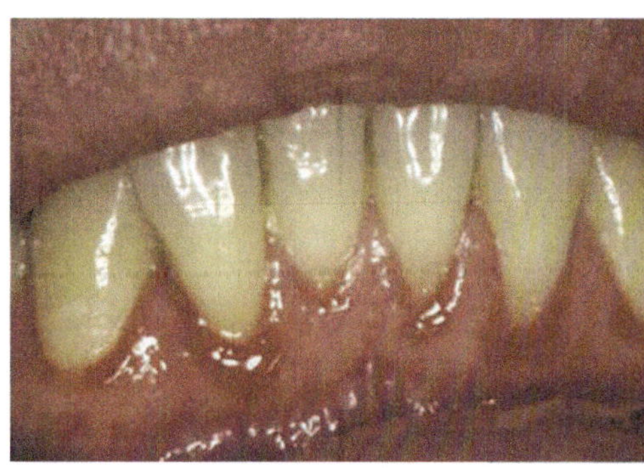

Fig. 12.1 HIV-infected patient with typical linear gingival erythema

periodontal disease under two groups, i.e. necrotizing ulcerative gingivitis (NUG) and necrotizing ulcerative periodontitis (NUP). A patient is considered to have LGE when there was a distinct, complete erythematous band present from papilla to adjacent papilla and extending at least 2 mm from the gingival margin. On the other hand, NUG patients have at least one papilla showing ulceration with a crater-like appearance and NUP has additional alveolar bone loss with at least 3 mm loss of attachment in the interproximal area. It has been shown that CD4+ T lymphocytes counting less than 500 and 200 cells/mm^3 are associated with NUG and NUP, respectively.

Most importantly, LGE is different from plaque-induced gingivitis as it does not correlate with the amount of plaque present in the disease sites (Umadevi et al. 2006). In the classical lesion, there is no ulceration and no pocketing or loss of attachments, which are associated with plaque-induced periodontal diseases. Hence, unlike NUG or NUP, LGE does not cause destructive consequence to the periodontium in HIV patients. However, it is difficult to comment on the prevalence of LGE and NUP in early studies due to the confusion of the terms as HIV-associated gingivitis and HIV-associated periodontitis without defining a proper clinical picture. Some may even consider LGE as the initial form of destructive periodontal disease in the HIV patients. It is possible that several overlapping disease conditions have been described as a common periodontal disease due to lack of clear definitions for different disease entities.

Microbiology of Linear Gingival Erythema

Microbiology of LGE has not been fully defined. However, studies with microbiological analysis of LGE and periodontal disease in HIV/AIDS patients in general should be interpreted with caution. The major problem of arriving at a conclusion for the associated microbiota with LGE is the method of sampling. Various sampling methods have been used in the studies that examine the microbiological aetiology of LGE. The studies that considered LGE as a variant of periodontal disease have commonly examined dental plaque samples obtained from the site of the lesions to correlate the pathogenic microbiota with LGE. On the other hand, studies looking into the oral candidiasis have taken samples such as gingival scraping, mouth rinse or saliva. This should be kept in mind when correlating the microbiological data derived from different studies with LGE. In addition, definition of the clinical picture of "LGE" is somewhat ambiguous among studies resulting in contradictory reports in the literature. Moreover, some have used pooled samples from different sites with no clear demarcation of supra or subgingival plaque whereas others have used a site-specific sampling. Culturing methods and identification techniques vary among studies. All foregoing factors preclude arriving at a firm conclusion of the microbiological aetiology of LGE.

Composition of the gingival microbiota in HIV patients and comparative healthy counterparts has also been investigated, although the results are diverse and somewhat contradictory in nature. Some report that HIV-positive and healthy subjects have similar microbial profiles whilst others show the opposite. Aas et al 2007 examined the subgingival plaque microbiota of HIV-positive patients in order to describe and compare the predominant bacterial and fungal species associated with gingivitis, periodontitis and LGE using 16S and 18S rDNA sequencing (Aas et al. 2007). Bacterial profile of the LGE was quite different from other disease entities. *Saccharomyces cerevisiae* was the only fungal species detected in the LGE samples. In contrast, periodontitis patients had predominant *Candida albicans*. Association of classical "red-complex" periodontal pathogens such as *Porphyromonas gingivalis*, *Tannerella forsythia* and *Treponema denticola* with periodontal diseases in HIV patients including LGE was not as strong as in the healthy counterparts. Interestingly, while classical periodontal pathogens were sparse, other unconventional species like *Gamella*, *Dialister*, *Streptococcus* and *Veillonella* were predominant in HIV patients. Hence, authors suggested that unconventional bacterial species rather than classical periodontal pathogens are involved in the periodontal disease of the subjects with HIV (Aas et al. 2007). Another study compared the composition of subgingival microbiota of HIV-seropositive patients under HAART therapy and HIV-seronegative subjects with chronic periodontitis using DNA probes and checkerboard assays (Goncalves et al. 2007). They found significant association of *Enterococcus faecalis* and *Acinetobacter baumannii* with the periodontal disease of HIV patients corroborating the foregoing idea that classical periodontal pathogens are not usually detected in the periodontitis of HIV patients. Early studies on LGE and NPD have also suggested an association with viral pathogens. Viruses such as Cytomegalovirus, Epstein–Barr virus, human herpes viruses and papillomavirus were proposed to play a role in the initiation and progression of LGE and NPD (Umadevi et al. 2006). However, these claims have not been backed up by substantial data to prove such as an association. HIV-infected patients are likely to develop infections of concurrent viral, bacterial and fungal infections. This holds true for the HIV-associated periodontal disease too. Therefore, it is possible that multiple pathogens contribute to the development of LGE and NUG/NUP. Presence of these uncommon bacterial species may be a reflection of the immune-compromised status of the patients that lead to colonization of atypical pathogens.

The famous EC-Clearinghouse classification of the oral lesions associated with HIV infection in 1993 (Table 12.1) categorized LGE as a separate disease entity under Group 1 oral diseases, i.e. lesions most commonly associated with HIV infection (Axéll et al. 1993; van der Waal 1997). Additionally, few variants of oral candidiasis such as pseudomembranous candidiasis, erythematous candidiasis and angular chelitis were also categorized under Group 1 (Table 12.1). Due to the omission of LGE as a candidiasis variant in the EC-Clearinghouse classification, most of the subsequent studies on oral candidiasis of HIV subjects had not examined LGE.

Later studies showed that LGE could be associated with *Candida* infection. It is noteworthy that almost all HIV subjects have a heavy candidal carriage, which does not necessarily imply they suffer from *Candida* infections. One study evaluated subgingival colonization of *Candida* between HIV-positive and HIV-negative subjects taking oral mucosal samples and subgingival samples (Lamster et al. 1998). Identification and characterization of *Candida* was performed by culture-dependent enumeration as well as DNA fingerprinting. Higher percentage of HIV-positive subjects had *Candida* in the subgingival samples and *Candida* titre tends to be higher among them compared to HIV-negative subjects. Interestingly, subgingival *Candida* had a unique DNA pattern different from mucosal *Candida* indicating that gingival *Candida* colonizers are not a contamination from mucosal colonizers. Hence, Lamster et al. (1998) suggested presence of *Candida* in the subgingival plaque of the HIV patients may have an aetiological contribution to the development of LGE lesion. There are other studies showing higher *Candida* carriage more than 50 % in the subgingival plaque samples of

Table 12.1 Oral manifestations associated with HIV infection according to the classification of EC Clearinghouse (1993)

Group 1: Lesions most commonly associated with HIV infection
Oral candidiasis
Erythematous candidiasis
Pseudomembranous candidiasis
Angular cheilitis
Oral hairy leukoplakia
Linear gingival erythema
Necrotizing gingivitis
Necrotizing periodontitis
Non-Hodgkin's lymphoma
Group 2: Lesions less commonly associated with HIV infection
Melanotic hyper-pigmentation
Ulcers not otherwise specified
Herpes simplex virus infection
Herpes zoster
Decreased salivary flow rate
Group 3: Lesions associated with HIV infection
Recurrent apthous ulcers
Molluscum contagiosum
Lichenoid reaction
Facial palsy
Erythema multiforme

HIV-infected patients suffering from HIV gingivitis (Zambon et al. 1990).

Grbic et al. (1995) examined the periodontal status of a cohort consisted of HIV-infected homosexual men and parenteral drug users with seronegative counterparts (Grbic et al. 1995). In addition, three variants of oral candidiasis, namely, pseudomembranous candidiasis, angular chelitis and erythematous candidiasis were also examined. Diagnosis of erythematous candidiasis was made from a smear taken from the erythematous area. Diagnosis criterion was presence of more than 10 hyphae of the lesion in Periodic Acid Schiff (PAS) stain. Interestingly, oral candidiasis as well as LGE was more prevalent in the subjects with decreased CD4+ lymphocytes. Hence, 42.9 % of the HIV-positive homosexual men having oral candidiasis had LGE whereas only 12.7 % of the subjects without candidiasis had LGE. Data from this study suggested a high likelihood of developing LGE in HIV-seropositive homosexuals if they have oral candidiasis. More interestingly, it was revealed, if the HIV patients had been treated with antifungals in the last 6 months, they are less likely to develop LGE, furnishing more evidence of candidal association with LGE.

Velegraki et al. (1999) demonstrated that LGE could be of candidal origin (Velegraki et al. 1999). By using CHORMagar and API32C methods, they identified *Candida albicans* in three paediatric HIV subjects and *C. dubliniensis* in one patient. Interesting, all lesions were healed upon treatment with antifungals showing a causal nature of *Candida* to LGE. Portela et al. in a series of studies on LGE demonstrated the possibility of *Candida* as the aetiological agent of LGE in HIV-infected patients. Subgingival plaque samples of HIV-infected children contained 42.3 % *Candida* species compared to 7.1 % HIV-negative children (Portela et al. 2004). *C. albicans* was the most commonly recovered species, but other non-*albicans* species such as *Candida dubliniensis*, *Candida glabrata* and *Candida tropicalis* and mixed species were also present in the subgingival plaque samples.

Another case report series evaluated the association of *Candida* with LGE in paediatric HIV patients, which were resistant to conventional plaque-removal therapy (Portela et al. 2012). They obtained the samples by frictionating a sterilized microbrush on the lesion (LGE) for mycological analysis. Subsequently, speciation of *Candida* was performed by CHROMagar Candida® and API 20C identification system demonstrating the presence of *Candida* in LGE lesions. All LGE lesions were successfully healed when treated with topical antifungal agents. This investigation provided strong evidence for the fungal aetiology of LGE in HIV-infected children. In another study of this group, *Candida* species such as *C. albicans*, *C. tropicalis* and *C. parapsilosis* were isolated from the saliva of HIV-infected children and upon the treatment with chlorhexidine gel the salivary candidal counts were significantly reduced, with the concomitant improvement of gingivitis (Machado et al. 2011). On the other hand, a study from Thai HIV-infected patients suggested that high prevalence of *Candida* in the periodontal pockets may be due to higher carriage of *Candida* in the saliva (Samaranayake et al. 2002). Serine proteases produced by the *Candida* isolated derived from LGE lesions in HIV patients have also been examined (Portela et al. 2010). It was found that SAPs secreted by *Candida* are able to cleave various components of host immune response and extracellular matrix proteins which facilitate the dissemination of *Candida* into deep organs protecting from the host immune response. In addition, histopathological studies on LGE lesions have observed *Candida* is able to penetrate the gingival epithelium in order to gain access to underlying soft tissues (Odden et al. 1994; Gomez et al. 1995). Therefore, there is substantial evidence to suggest a strong association of *Candida* with the LGE lesion seen in HIV-infected subjects.

Prevalence of LGE in HIV-Infected Patients

HIV-infected patients are medically complex subjects. Therefore, prevalence of an oral manifestation like LGE may have many confounding factors. Patients' data such as age, status of HIV infection, oral hygiene status, other medical

Table 12.2 Prevalence of LGE and its association with oral candidiasis

Year	Population (mean age)	Country	Prevalence of LGE	Commonest oral disease (prevalence)	Reference
1991	Adults (33)	USA	75 % (LGE not)	Not examined	Klein et al. 1991
1994	Adults (40/41 %)	USA	16.1 % (homosexual) and drug users 33.3 %	Oral candidiasis (17.3) and 43 %	Lamster et al. 1994
2000	Mixed (33)	USA	3.30 %	Pseudomembranous candidiasis (12 %)	Patton et al. 2000
2001	Children (8.8)	Italy	4.00 %	Candidiasis (29 %)	Flaitz et al. 2001
2001	Adults (31.3)	Thailand	8 %	Pseudomembranous candidiasis (10.3 %)	Khongkunthian et al. 2001
2001	Adults (31.9)	Thailand	11.50 %	Pseudomembranous candidiasis (39.6 %)	Nittayananta et al. 2001
2003	Children (5.5)	Thailand	20 %	Oral candidiasis (45 %)	Pongsiriwet et al. 2003
2008	Adults (38.3)	South India	11.50 %	Erythematous candidiasis (44 %)	Sharma et al. 2009
2008	Adults	Nigeria	24 %	Pseudomembranous candidiasis (43.1 %)	Adedigba et al. 2008
2008	Adults (35.4)	Ethiopia	12 %	Pseudomembraneous candidiasis (20.1 %)	Guteta et al. 2008
2010	Adults (39)	Brazil	22	Oral candidiasis (49 %)	Aleixo et al. 2010
2010	Adults (35.6)	Nigeria	0.70 %	Pseudomembranous candidiasis (6.3 %)	Taiwo et al. 2010
2011	Mixed (33)	India	2.40 %	Pseudomembraneous candidiasis (20.1 %)	Sontakke et al. 2011
2011	Adults	Iran	22.00 %	Linear gingival erythema (22 %)	Khatibi et al. 2011
2011	Mixed (33)	India	10.30 %	Erythematous candidiasis (30.6 %)	Bodhade et al. 2011
2012	Adults (34)	India	45.50 %	Not examined	Ranganathan et al. 2012
2012	Adults (47.38)	USA	3	Oral candidiasis (24.2)	Freeman et al. 2012
2003	Children (7.7)	USA	22	Oral candidiasis 38 %	Fine et al. 2003
2010	Children (7.09)	South Africa	<5 %	Oral candidiasis (65.5 %)	Duggal et al. 2010
2013	Adults (32.4)	Nepal	17.30 %	Oral candidiasis (21 %)	Naidu et al. 2013
2013	Children (5.74)	Brazil	15.30 %	Gingivitis (84.6 %)	A. de Aguiar Ribeiro et al. 2013

problems, use of medication such as HAART and antimicrobials may significantly affect the presence of oral diseases including LGE in HIV-infected patients. In addition, definition of the clinical diagnosis, experience of the clinician, whether the diagnosis was purely of clinical basis or accompanied with microbiological and histopathological assays all affect the final diagnosis of the disease. Even in the post-HAART era, different institutions use various combinations of the anti-retroviral drugs; hence, these data cannot be directly compared. Unfortunately not all studies have clearly mentioned that information in their study cohorts. In addition, most of the studies in the literature on LGE are cross-sectional in nature. This paucity essentially precludes a proper comparison of the disease and data on the prevalence must be analysed with parsimony. Nevertheless, prevalence of the LGE in these past studies provides a general trend of the LGE in HIV patients (Table 12.2).

Prevalence of LGE reported to be ranging from 0 to 92 % (Khongkunthian et al. 2001; Miziara et al. 2006; Guteta et al. 2008; Aleixo et al. 2010; Sontakke et al. 2011). As LGE was not categorized under variant of oral candidiasis in EC-Clearinghouse classification (Axéll et al. 1993), data of the prevalence of LGE mostly come from the studies that examined the periodontal diseases of the HIV patients or studies that generally look into all oral manifestations.

In general, introduction of HAART has also reduced the incidence of oral lesions including LGE and oral candidiasis in adults (Kroidl et al. 2005). On the contrary, HAART does not appear to significantly affect the prevalence of periodontal disease in children (de Aguiar Ribeiro et al. 2013). Emerging data from new studies indicate HIV/AIDS patients in post-HAART ears are likely to develop AIDS-associated infections including oral candidiasis in some point of their life.

HAART agents such as zidovudine, nevirapine have reduced the oral candidiasis due to two major reasons. First, immune reconstitution increases the number of the CD4+ and CD8+ T cells enhancing patient's host defence against *Candida* infection. Second, unexpectedly, it was discovered that HAART possesses a protease inhibitory action: secretary aspartyl proteases of *Candida*. Secretary aspartyl proteases or SAPs are considered a major virulence attribute of *Candida* that facilitates the tissue invasion (Portela et al. 2010). Therefore, reduction of LGE in post-HAART era may also be due to the suppression of SAPs of *Candida*. On the other hand, some studies have shown that HAART has reduced the pseudomembranous and hyperplastic variants of candidiasis in HIV patients whilst prevalence of erythematous candidiasis has increased (Ceballos-Salobrena et al. 2004). Some recent studies have shown that oral candidiasis is still the predominant oral manifestation of the HIV/AIDS status of HIV-infected paediatric patients who are under HARRT therapy (Nesti et al. 2012).

In an early study, Klein et al 1991 reported the higher percentage (85 %) of HIV-associated gingivitis and periodontitis among heterosexual subjects (Klein et al. 1991). Out of the patients who had HIV-gingivitis as the sole manifestation of periodontal disease, 59 % had involvement of all quadrants. It is noteworthy that the patients with HIV-gingivitis in this study had features like marked oedema and erythema of the gingiva, pain, spontaneous bleeding, interproximal necrosis and ulceration. Therefore, it is likely that HIV-gingivitis reported in this study may reflect a combined clinical picture of LGE and NUG. Therefore, exact percentage of patients with LGE cannot be accurately determined.

Interestingly, a recent retrospective study performed in Adelaide Dental Hospital analysing the oral lesions of HIV patients on HAART noted that combined anti-retroviral therapy may have increased LGE of patients compared to mono-HAART therapy (Freeman et al. 2012). Oral candidiasis was the second most common oral lesion amongst the cohort. Pseudomembranous variant was the commonest, followed by erythematous candidiasis. It has to be noted that other confounding factors such as presence of dry mouth and comorbidities such as diabetes mellitus or asthma may have partly contributed to the enhancement of candidiasis in these patients. Another recent study conducted on the Iranian patients have shown a 16.5 % prevalence of LGE and 22 % of oral candidiasis as oral manifestations of HIV AIDS patients (Khatibi et al. 2011). A Taiwan study reported a presence of 5.8 % of LGE and 12.1 % of oral candidiasis in HIV-infected patients (Chiang et al. 1998). Analysis of Chinese cohort of 203 HIV/AIDS patients showed that oral candidiasis is the most common lesion (66 %) and LGE is to be 2 % (Zhang et al. 2009). Study on HIV-positive Indian patients found that erythematous candidiasis (44 %), linear gingival erythema (11.5 %) and pseudomembranous candidiasis (10.5 %) were the common oral findings (Sharma et al. 2009). Another study on Indian cohort reported that 10.27 % of 399 HIV-positive patients had LGE (Bodhade et al. 2011). In addition, a recent study in Nigerian HIV patients not under HAART reconfirmed the predominant presence of oral candidiasis (Adedigba et al. 2008). The commonest HIV lesion was pseudomembranous candidiasis (43.1 %) followed by erythematous candidiasis (28.9 %), angular cheilitis (28.9 %) and linear gingival erythema (24 %). In contrast, another study on Nigerian HIV patients taking HAART reported very low level (0.7 %) of LGE and 6.5 % of oral candidiasis (Taiwo and Hassan 2010).

LGE was also shown to be a significant problem among HIV-infected children in some studies whereas others report to be a minor problem (Barasch et al. 2000; Fonseca et al. 2000; Schoen et al. 2000; Flaitz et al. 2001; Fine et al. 2003; Pongsiriwet et al. 2003; Nesti et al. 2012) Studies on paediatric HIV patients in various countries have reported the presence of LGE to be in the range from 0 to 48 % (Ramos-Gomez 2002). However, it is well known that oral candidiasis is the most common oral lesion associated with paediatric HIV patients (Ramos-Gomez 2002; Coogan et al. 2005). It seems that HAART may have a lesser effect on LGE and oral candidiasis in paediatric patients compared to adult HIV patients (Coogan et al. 2005).

Diagnosis and Treatment

By definition, LGE is neither associated with the amount of plaque present at the gingival sites nor responds well to plaque management (Umadevi et al. 2006). However, if there is a need, periodontal treatment in the form of scaling and root debridement is advisable (Phelan 1997; Hofer et al. 2002). Chemical plaque control by means of a mouthwash containing 0.12 % of chlorhexidine for 2 weeks has been used for treating LGE lesions. Chlorhexidine is a widely used antimicrobial agent for maintaining oral health as well as treatment purpose for oral infections. Topical application of chlorhexidine has also been used as an antifungal agent. A study evaluated the efficacy of 0.2 % CHX gel on HIV-infected children (Machado et al. 2011). The children were instructed to brush their teeth with the gel for 1 min twice a day over 21 days and not to use fluoride dentifrice or dental floss during this period. After the study period, it was noted that 73 % reduction in gingivitis as well as 68 % reduction of candidal carriage. This provides evidence that *Candida* carriage may have an association with the gingivitis (LGE) seen in HIV patients.

Diagnosis of the oral *Candida* lesion in general could be done by culture, smear and biopsy. Serial sections biopsies may demonstrate the presence of candidal hyphae in the epithelium. Mild epithelial dysplasia may accompany the fungal invasion. However, it should be born in mind that *Candida* carriage is common among people including healthy subjects. Therefore, microbiological findings and compatible clinical features should be taken into consideration before arriving at a diagnosis. For instance, presence of hyphae or pseudohyphae is a good indication of the tissue penetration of *Candida* in the gingiva, which has been shown in the LGE lesion of HIV-infected patients (Odden et al. 1994).

The American Academy of Periodontology considers LGE as a gingival disease of fungal origin (Armitage 1999). If LGE does not respond well to plaque control measures, antifungal treatment should be initiated immediately. Drug–drug interaction should be born in mind when prescribing antifungal agents such as fluconazole, ketoconazole and itraconazole as they may interact with the antiretroviral therapy as well as other antimicrobials (Phelan 1997). For instance, azole agent ketoconazole may interact with AZT (zidovudine) as both use cytochrome-C cellular system for metabolism. In addition, effectiveness of ketoconazole may be reduced by rifampin, a drug used to treat tuberculosis (Phelan 1997).

Considering the foregoing information, it could be concluded that administration of topical antifungal agent or antimicrobial agent like 0.2 % chlorhexidine may be beneficial for the patients with LGE. Whether it is due to effect on pathogenic *Candida* species present in the sites or due to general effect on improving healthy dental plaque biofilm or salivary microbiota remains to be fully elucidated.

Proposed Mechanism

Oral epithelial cells and gingival epithelial cells play an important role as the first line of host innate immune defence against various microorganisms including *Candida*. Upon recognition of the invading *Candida* species, epithelial cells secrete antimicrobial peptides such as β-defensins and various cytokines to resist and clear the *Candida* invasion (Cheng et al. 2012). Polymorphonuclear leucocytes, in particular neutrophils, are important to control the *Candida* invasion of epithelial tissues (Naglik et al. 2011). It has been shown that polymorphonuclear leucocyte activity and chemotaxis are impaired in HIV/AIDS (Shalekoff et al. 1998; Hofman et al. 1999). CD88 expression of PMNL has been shown to be defective in AIDS state. These factors may contribute to the high prevalence of oral *Candida* lesions seen in HIV-infected patients including that of LGE (Goncalves et al. 2013).

Pathogenesis of LGE seemed to be multifactorial representing both host as well as microbial factors. HIV infection has a larger bearing on the appearance of LGE. For instance, as mentioned above, reduced CD4+ T cells have weakened the host adaptive immune as well as probably the innate immune responses. The oral lesions of HIV infection in general are opportunistic and their presence is somewhat correlated with the viral load and CD4+ cell counts. Moreover, significant inverse relationship of LGE with CD4+ cell numbers has been observed, which shows its reliability as an indicator for immune suppression (Ranganathan et al. 2012). High viral load and the low CD4 cell counts have been shown to be correlated with the oral manifestations LGE of HIV-infected children as well. It is noteworthy that immune reconstitution, i.e. increased number CD4+ and CD8+ T cells due to HAART therapy has markedly reduced the *Candida* infections in HIV patients in general (Reichart 2003; Coogan et al. 2005; Mataftsi et al. 2011). Based on these findings, low CD4+ counts are now considered as the main risk factors associated with the development of oral lesions and especially of oral candidiasis (Margiotta et al. 1999). LGE has a significant predictive value (70 %) for immune suppression when measured by CD4 cell counts below 200 cells mm (Patton 2000). Therefore, presence of LGE has been suggested as a predictor of the progression of the HIV infections towards AIDS (Begg et al. 1997; Coogan et al. 2005).

Some light on the pathogenic mechanism of LGE has been shed by the histopathological studies examining the LGE (Gomez et al. 1995; Lamster et al. 1998). The relative population of T-lymphocytes, B-lymphocytes, macrophages, neutrophils and IgG bearing plasma cells has been compared in the gingival biopsies obtained from sites exhibiting LGE with biopsies from non-specific gingivitis (Gomez et al. 1995). LGE biopsies had an increased level of neutrophils and IgG plasma cells whilst decreased level of T cell and macrophages compared to the biopsies from non-specific gingivitis. Presence of intraepithelial neutrophils in the gingival epithelium was also observed in the gingival biopsies of LGE patients. They proposed that influx of polymorphonuclear leucocytes (PMN) contributes to the lesion seen in LGE.

Another study compared the gingival biopsies taken from 27 HIV seropositive subjects who had gingival manifestations with HIV-seronegative subjects with periodontitis (Odden et al. 1994). Candidal hyphae and pseudohyphae were found in the parakeratinized oral epithelium in HIV-infected patients whereas no fungal invasion was found in any of the biopsies from the HIV-seronegative subjects. Heavy polymorphonuclear leucocyte infiltration of the oral gingival epithelium accompanied by acanthosis and intracellular oedema was observed in response to candidial invasion. This study also provided a strong association of *Candida* with LGE in HIV patients (Odden, Schenck et al. 1994).

Analysis of GCF components from the HIV-infected subjects of various origins (sexual transmission and drug users) has shown that both groups possess comparable immune response such as PMN-derived lysosomal enzyme ß-glucuronidase, IgA and IgM (Grbic et al. 1997). Evaluated level of IL-1β and IgG has been observed in HIV-positive subjects. It is worthwhile to examine the effect of salivary defence in the HIV status in general. However, the present understanding is it might not be a critical factor in the HIV-associated oral candidiasis as mucosal IgA and IgG are intact.

Hyphal invasion of *Candida* may evoke a local immune-inflammatory response, thereby inducing excessive secretion of host inflammatory markers such as metalloproteinases, IL-6, IL-8 and IL-1β in the periodontal pockets of HIV patients. This may trigger the excessive infiltration of neutrophils to the site of lesion causing a cycle of inflammatory response. All these factors together contribute to the changes in the gingival tissues as seen in LGE and NUG/NUP and may lead to chronic periodontal diseases of the HIV/AIDS patients.

Conclusion and Future Directions

Considering the foregoing information, it could be concluded that there is a strong association of *Candida* as an aetiological agent for LGE in HIV-infected patients. Although LGE as well as other oral infections including oral candidiasis may have reduced with the introduction of HAART, still the prevalence of LGE is considerable, in particular among paediatric HIV patients. Therefore, clinicians should be vigilant of the LGE in HIV patients in order to diagnose the condition and for early therapeutic intervention. Although there is no conclusive evidence to suggest antifungal treatment for all patients with LGE, antifungals as a therapeutic option should be considered in appropriate cases. More studies into the incidence of LGE in HIV patients, in particular who are under HAART, are warranted. Clinical studies demonstrating the therapeutic intervention to the lesions as well as careful and comprehensive analysis of the dental plaque samples using newer molecular biological techniques will shed more light on the pathogenesis and treatment of LGE in HIV patients.

References

Aas JA, Barbuto SM, Alpagot T, Olsen I, Dewhirst FE, Paster BJ (2007) Subgingival plaque microbiota in HIV positive patients. J Clin Periodontol 34(3):189–195

Adedigba MA, Ogunbodede EO, Jeboda SO, Naidoo S (2008) Patterns of oral manifestation of HIV/AIDS among 225 Nigerian patients. Oral Dis 14(4):341–346

Aleixo RQ, Scherma AP, Guimaraes G, Cortelli JR, Cortelli SC (2010) DMFT index and oral mucosal lesions associated with HIV infection: cross-sectional study in Porto Velho, Amazonian region – Brazil. Braz J Infect Dis 14(5):449–456

Armitage GC (1999) Development of a classification system for periodontal diseases and conditions. Ann Periodontol 4(1):1–6

Axéll T, Azuln AM, Challacombet SJ, Ficarra G, Flint S, Greenspan D, Hammerle C, Laskaris G, Loeb I, Lucas-Tomas M, Monteil RA, Pindborg JJ, Riechart P, Robinson P, Scully C, Swango P, Syrjnen S, Thornhill MH, van der Waal I, Williams DM, Wray D (1993) Classification and diagnostic criteria for oral lesions in HIV infection. EC-clearinghouse on oral problems related to HIV infection and WHO collaborating centre on oral manifestations of the immunodeficiency virus. J Oral Pathol Med 22(7):289–291

Barasch A, Safford MM, Catalanotto FA, Fine DH, Katz RV (2000) Oral soft tissue manifestations in HIV-positive vs. HIV-negative children from an inner city population: a two-year observational study. Pediatr Dent 22(3):215–220

Begg MD, Lamster IB, Panageas KS, Mitchell-Lewis D, Phelan JA, Grbic JT (1997) A prospective study of oral lesions and their predictive value for progression of HIV disease. Oral Dis 3(3):176–183

Bodhade AS, Ganvir SM, Hazarey VK (2011) Oral manifestations of HIV infection and their correlation with CD4 count. J Oral Sci 53(2):203–211

Ceballos-Salobrena A, Gaitain-Cepeda L, Ceballos-Garcia L, Samaranayake LP (2004) The effect of antiretroviral therapy on the prevalence of HIV-associated oral candidiasis in a Spanish cohort. Oral Surg Oral Med Oral Pathol Oral Radiol Endod 97(3):345–350

Cerqueira DF, Portela MB, Pomarico L, de Araujo Soares RM, de Souza IP, Castro GF (2010) Oral Candida colonization and its relation with predisposing factors in HIV-infected children and their uninfected siblings in Brazil: the era of highly active antiretroviral therapy. J Oral Pathol Med 39(2):188–194

Cheng SC, Joosten LA, Kullberg BJ, Netea MG (2012) Interplay between Candida albicans and the mammalian innate host defense. Infect Immun 80(4):1304–1313

Chiang CP, Chueh LH, Lin SK, Chen MY (1998) Oral manifestations of human immunodeficiency virus-infected patients in Taiwan. J Formos Med Assoc 97(9):600–605

Coogan MM, Greenspan J, Challacombe SJ (2005) Oral lesions in infection with human immunodeficiency virus. Bull World Health Organ 83(9):700–706

de Aguiar Ribeiro A, Portela MB, de Souza IP (2013) The oral health of HIV infected Brazilian children. Int J Paediatr Dent 23(5):359–365

Duggal MS, Abudiak H, Dunn C, Tong HJ, Munyombwe T (2010) Effect of CD4+ lymphocyte count, viral load, and duration of taking anti-retroviral treatment on presence of oral lesions in a sample of South African children with HIV+/AIDS. Eur Arch Paediatr Dent 11(5):242–6

Fine DH, Tofsky N, Nelson EM, Schoen D, Barasch A (2003) Clinical implications of the oral manifestations of HIV infection in children. Dent Clin North Am 47(1):159–174, xi-xii

Flaitz C, Wullbrandt B, Sexton J, Bourdon T, Hicks J (2001) Prevalence of orodental findings in HIV-infected Romanian children. Pediatr Dent 23(1):44–50

Fonseca R, Cardoso AS, Pomarico I (2000) Frequency of oral manifestations in children infected with human immunodeficiency virus. Quintessence Int 31(6):419–422

Freeman AD, Liberali SA, Coates EA, Logan RM (2012) Oral health in Australian HIV patients since the advent of combination antiretroviral therapy. Aust Dent J 57(4):470–476, quiz 518

Gomez RS, da Costa JE, Loyola AM, de Araujo NS, de Araujo VC (1995) Immunohistochemical study of linear gingival erythema from HIV-positive patients. J Periodontal Res 30(5):355–359

Goncalves LS, Soares Ferreira SM, Souza CO, Souto R, Colombo AP (2007) Clinical and microbiological profiles of human immunodeficiency virus (HIV)-seropositive Brazilians undergoing highly active antiretroviral therapy and HIV-seronegative Brazilians with chronic periodontitis. J Periodontol 78(1):87–96

Goncalves LS, Goncalves BM, Fontes TV (2013) Periodontal disease in HIV-infected adults in the HAART era: clinical, immunological, and microbiological aspects. Arch Oral Biol 58(10):1385–1396

Grbic JT, Mitchell-Lewis DA, Fine JB, Phelan JA, Bucklan RS, Zambon JJ, Lamster IB (1995) The relationship of candidiasis to linear gingival erythema in HIV-infected homosexual men and parenteral drug users. J Periodontol 66(1):30–37

Grbic JT, Lamster IB, Mitchell-Lewis D (1997) Inflammatory and immune mediators in crevicular fluid from HIV-infected injecting drug users. J Periodontol 68(3):249–255

Guteta S, Feleke Y, Fekade D, Neway M, Diro E (2008) Prevalence of oral and perioral manifestations in HIV positive adults at Tikur Anbessa Teaching Hospital Addis Ababa, Ethiopia. Ethiop Med J 46(4):349–357

Hofer D, Hammerle CH, Grassi M, Lang NP (2002) Long-term results of supportive periodontal therapy (SPT) in HIV-seropositive and HIV-seronegative patients. J Clin Periodontol 29(7):630–637

Hofman P, Fischer F, Far DF, Selva E, Battaglione V, Bayle J, Rossi B (1999) Impairment of HIV polymorphonuclear leukocyte transmigration across T84 cell monolayers: an alternative mechanisms for increased intestinal bacterial infections in AIDS? Eur Cytokine Netw 10(3):373–382

Khatibi M, Moshari AA, Jahromi ZM, Ramezankhani A (2011) Prevalence of oral mucosal lesions and related factors in 200 HIV+/AIDS Iranian patients. J Oral Pathol Med 40(8):659–664

Khongkunthian P, Grote M, Isaratanan W, Plyaworawong S, Reichart PA (2001) Oral manifestations in HIV-positive adults from Northern Thailand. J Oral Pathol Med 30(4):220–223

Klein RS, Quart AM, Small CB (1991) Periodontal disease in heterosexuals with acquired immunodeficiency syndrome. J Periodontol 62(8):535–540

Kroidl A, Schaeben A, Oette M, Wettstein M, Herfordt A, Haussinger D (2005) Prevalence of oral lesions and periodontal diseases in HIV-infected patients on antiretroviral therapy. Eur J Med Res 10(10):448–453

Lamster IB, Begg MD, Mitchell-Lewis D, Fine JB, Grbic JT, Todak GG, el-Sadr W, Gorman JM, Zambon JJ, Phelan JA (1994) Oral manifestations of HIV infection in homosexual men and intravenous drug users. Study design and relationship of epidemiologic, clinical, and immunologic parameters to oral lesions. Oral Surg Oral Med Oral Pathol 78(2):163–174

Lamster IB, Grbic JT, Mitchell-Lewis DA, Begg MD, Mitchell A (1998) New concepts regarding the pathogenesis of periodontal disease in HIV infection. Ann Periodontol 3(1):62–75

Machado FC, de Souza IP, Portela MB, de Araujo Soares RM, Freitas-Fernandes LB, Castro GF (2011) Use of chlorhexidine gel (0.2%) to control gingivitis and candida species colonization in human immunodeficiency virus-infected children: a pilot study. Pediatr Dent 33(2):153–157

Margiotta V, Campisi G, Mancuso S, Accurso V, Abbadessa V (1999) HIV infection: oral lesions, CD4+ cell count and viral load in an Italian study population. J Oral Pathol Med 28(4):173–177

Mataftsi M, Skoura L, Sakellari D (2011) HIV infection and periodontal diseases: an overview of the post-HAART era. Oral Dis 17(1):13–25

Miziara ID, Filho BC, Weber R (2006) Oral lesions in Brazilian HIV-infected children undergoing HAART. Int J Pediatr Otorhinolaryngol 70(6): 1089–1096

Naglik JR, Moyes DL, Wachtler B, Hube B (2011) Candida albicans interactions with epithelial cells and mucosal immunity. Microbes Infect 13(12-13): 963–976

Naidu GS, Thakur R, Singh AK, Rajbhandary S, Mishra RK, Sagtani A (2013) Oral lesions and immune status of HIV infected adults from eastern Nepal. J Clin Exp Dent 5(1):e1–7

Nesti M, Carli E, Giaquinto C, Rampon O, Nastasio S, Giuca MR (2012) Correlation between viral load, plasma levels of CD4–CD8 T lymphocytes and AIDS-related oral diseases: a multicentre study on 30 HIV+ children in the HAART era. J Biol Regul Homeost Agents 26(3):527–537

Nittayananta W, Chanowanna N, Sripatanakul S, Winn T (2001) Risk factors associated with oral lesions in HIV-infected heterosexual people and intravenous drug users in Thailand. J Oral Pathol Med 30(4):224–230

Odden K, Schenck K, Koppang H, Hurlen B (1994) Candidal infection of the gingiva in HIV-infected persons. J Oral Pathol Med 23(4):178–183

Patton LL (2000) Sensitivity, specificity, and positive predictive value of oral opportunistic infections in adults with HIV/AIDS as markers of immune suppression and viral burden. Oral Surg Oral Med Oral Pathol Oral Radiol Endod 90(2):182–188

Phelan JA (1997) Dental lesions: diagnosis and treatment. Oral Dis 3(Suppl 1):S235–S237

Pongsiriwet S, Iamaroon A, Kanjanavanit S, Pattanaporn K, Krisanaprakornkit S (2003) Oral lesions and dental caries status in perinatally HIV-infected children in Northern Thailand. Int J Paediatr Dent 13(3): 180–185

Portela MB, Souza IP, Costa EM, Hagler AN, Soares RM, Santos AL (2004) Differential recovery of Candida species from subgingival sites in human immunodeficiency virus-positive and healthy children from Rio de Janeiro, Brazil. J Clin Microbiol 42(12):5925–5927

Portela MB, Souza IP, Abreu CM, Bertolini M, Holandino C, Alviano CS, Santos AL, Soares RM (2010) Effect of serine-type protease of Candida spp. isolated from linear gingival erythema of HIV-positive children: critical factors in the colonization. J Oral Pathol Med 39(10):753–760

Portela MS, de Cerqueira DFM, Araujo S, Castro GF (2012) Candida spp. in linear gingival erythema lesions in HIV-infected children: reports of six cases. Inter J Sci Dentist 51–55

Ramos-Gomez F (2002) Dental considerations for the paediatric AIDS/HIV patient. Oral Dis 8(Suppl 2):49–54

Ranganathan AT, Saraswathi PK, Albert V, Baba MG, Panishankar KH (2012) Route of transmission might influence the clinical expression of periodontal lesions in "human immunodeficiency virus" positive patients. Niger J Clin Pract 15(3):349–353

Reichart PA (2003) Oral manifestations in HIV infection: fungal and bacterial infections, Kaposi's sarcoma. Med Microbiol Immunol 192(3):165–169

Reznik DA (2005) Oral manifestations of HIV disease. Top HIV Med 13(5):143–148

Ryder MI, Nittayananta W, Coogan M, Greenspan D, Greenspan JS (2012) Periodontal disease in HIV/AIDS. Periodontol 2000 60(1):78–97

Samaranayake LP, Fidel PL, Naglik JR, Sweet SP, Teanpaisan R, Coogan MM, Blignaut E, Wanzala P (2002) Fungal infections associated with HIV infection. Oral Dis 8(Suppl 2):151–160

Samaranayake LP, Keung Leung W, Jin L (2009) Oral mucosal fungal infections. Periodontol 2000(49): 39–59

Schoen DH, Murray PA, Nelson E, Catalanotto FA, Katz RV, Fine DH (2000) A comparison of periodontal disease in HIV-infected children and household peers: a two year report. Pediatr Dent 22(5):365–369

Shalekoff S, Tiemessen CT, Gray CM, Martin DJ (1998) Depressed phagocytosis and oxidative burst in polymorphonuclear leukocytes from individuals with pulmonary tuberculosis with or without human immunodeficiency virus type 1 infection. Clin Diagn Lab Immunol 5(1):41–44

Sharma G, Pai KM, Setty S, Ramapuram JT, Nagpal A (2009) Oral manifestations as predictors of immune suppression in a HIV-/AIDS-infected population in south India. Clin Oral Investig 13(2):141–148

Sontakke SA, Umarji HR, Karjodkar F (2011) Comparison of oral manifestations with CD4 count in HIV-infected patients. Indian J Dent Res 22(5):732

Taiwo OO, Hassan Z (2010) The impact of highly active antiretroviral therapy (HAART) on the clinical features of HIV-related oral lesions in Nigeria. AIDS Res Ther 7:19

Umadevi M, Adeyemi O, Patel M, Reichart PA, Robinson PG (2006) (B2) Periodontal diseases and other bacterial infections. Adv Dent Res 19(1):139–145

van der Waal I (1997) Some unusual oral lesions in HIV infection: comments on the current classification. Oral Dis 3(Suppl 1):S197–S199

Velegraki A, Nicolatou O, Theodoridou M, Mostrou G, Legakis NJ (1999) Paediatric AIDS–related linear gingival erythema: a form of erythematous candidiasis? J Oral Pathol Med 28(4):178–182

Winkler JR, Murray PA (1987) Periodontal disease. A potential intraoral expression of AIDS may be rapidly progressive periodontitis. CDA J 15(1):20–24

Zambon JJ, Reynolds HS, Genco RJ (1990) Studies of the subgingival microflora in patients with acquired immunodeficiency syndrome. J Periodontol 61(11): 699–704

Zhang X, Reichart PA, Song Y (2009) Oral manifestations of HIV/AIDS in China: a review. Oral Maxillofac Surg 13(2):63–68

Index

E.A.R. Rosa (ed.), *Oral Candidosis: Physiopathology, Decision Making, and Therapeutics,*
DOI 10.1007/978-3-662-47194-4

9783662471937